COVID-19

AFRICA, HAITI, AND THE U. S. VIRGIN ISLANDS:

The Response, the Aftermath, & Future Projections

HUGUES FIDELE BATSIELILIT, PH. D.

Public Health Specialist

COVID-19: Africa, Haiti, and the U.S. Virgin Islands: The Response, the Aftermath, & Future Projections

Please send all correspondence to:

The International Consulting Aid Network (ICAN)

609 Gravlee Lane

Birmingham, Alabama, 35206

AUTHOR

Dr. Hugues Fidele Batsielilit, Ph.D., is the President and CEO of the International Consulting Aid Network (ICAN). He worked as an emergency management specialist focusing on health, public health issues, and post-disaster impacts (Federal Emergency Management Agency), served as an expert international consultant in public health surveillance, a communicable disease specialist (The Peace Corps, and ICAN), a healthcare administrator, and a community health coordinator for more than ten years.

Batsielilit received his Bachelor of Science degree from the National Institute of Executives, a Master of Sciences and a Ph.D. in public health and healthcare administration from the University of Phoenix in Arizona. Additionally, Dr. Batsielilit holds an associate degree in medical logistics from the Fort Lee Military Academy in Virginia. He served in the United States Army from 2008 to 2012, where he was assigned to the 82nd Airborne Medical Division as a medical logistics specialist.

Dr. Batsielilit is a member of several professional associations, including the Army Medical Veterans, the Peace Corps RPCV, the Nonprofit Association of Alabama, the Red Cross, the Birmingham Chamber of Commerce, the British Council, and the American College of Healthcare Executives.

PREFACE

The novel coronavirus - COVID-19 - that took the world by storm and was first seen in Wuhan Province, China, in December 2019, saw what appeared to be its first remission by June 2020. While nations around the world were reopening, developing countries, especially in Africa, the USVI, and Haiti, were still experiencing increasing rates of severe COVID-19infection.

As per experts, the severity and continued pathology were, (and remain), because of the virus's ability to attack people of all age groups. It is especially virulent among those with pre-existing medical conditions such as cardiovascular disease, conventional cardiovascular risk factors, diabetes, obesity, hypertension, malnutrition, other infectious diseases, and malaria – all of which are persistent in Africa and Haiti. While it remains rampant in these areas, scientists are still learning about COVID-19 and how it affects people with HIV/AIDS. This population, with weakened immune systems, is a prime target for the prolific virus. HIV/AIDS and the pre-existing medical conditions mentioned all require professional routinely monitored medical care.

With many countries now in various stages of quarantine,

fewer people are going to health facilities, which implies even fewer individuals are receiving the critical care or medicine they should, whether they have HIV, need vaccinations for their children, or prenatal care.

This is all rendered poorer by the failure of health systems and insufficient services and capacity (intensive care units, hospital beds, and specialized equipment), especially in remote and rural localities.

Overpopulation in informal urban communities and displaced refugee camps, and the absence of access to clean water and sanitation also engender attractive conditions for COVID-19 to thrive and spread at an alarming rate. By July 12, 2020, there were over 12,322.395 million confirmed cases with 556,335 deaths in 216 countries or territories, according to the World Health Organization (WHO).[1]

Until the appearance of COVID-19 in late 2019, most people had not heard of coronaviruses. However, this class of viruses and the infections they cause in humans and animals were first seen fifty-five years ago in 1965.

In 1965, Almeida and Tyrel, with six other colleagues, identified several types of coronaviruses - a group of viruses "that caused not only avian bronchitis but also murine hepatitis and upper respiratory tract diseases in human beings."[2] The scientists categorized the strain that caused avian infectious bronchitis as a gamma coronavirus, while most coronaviruses that affect humans are beta coronaviruses.

The various strains of corona viruses can cause a broad scope of infections, from mild, resembling the common cold, to harmful illnesses such as Severe Acute Respiratory Syndrome (SARS), (also known as SARS-CoV), and Middle East Respiratory Syndrome (MERS), (also known as MERS-CoV).

A strain of coronavirus analogous to SARS-CoV, the strain that triggered the 2003 SARS pandemic (described in the following chapters) also triggered the COVID-19 pandemic. There has been speculation that the current pandemic coronavirus results from an unintentional lab accident wherein bat coronaviruses were released; however, this has not been substantiated. [3-5]

Like the circumstances of the first reported incidence of COVID-19, it is significant to highlight that during the 2003 SARS pandemic, which also occurred in China, the Chinese authorities did not cooperate with the WHO in sharing information about the disease event for four months. This resulted in delayed assistance and research that may have been beneficial in stemming the transmission of the virus which, according to the WHO, ravaged the lives of 8,347 people across 5 continents, with 813 deaths.[6]

Reluctance to provide critical disease incidence information led to the WHO requesting the International Health Regulations Board establish regulations and reforms on how nations cope with public health disasters and guidelines on the reporting of outbreaks. In the current pandemic environment, there are still questions surrounding the root of the SARS-CoV-2 virus known to trigger COVID-19.

It has been determined that SARS resulted from infection caused by a coronavirus called SARS-associated coronavirus (SARS-CoV). This specific virus is linked to the novel severe acute respiratory syndrome coronavirus 2 (SARS-CoV-2). Although COVID-19 is an ongoing worldwide challenge, no evidence of new occurrences of SARS have emerged since 2004, and it may take many years to discover a virus in animals matching SARS-CoV-2.

TABLE OF CONTENTS

CHAPTER ONE

Origin and Global History of COVID-19

Literature Evaluation Methodology

An evaluation of existing literature that defines the prevailing state of COVID-19 in the nations of African, the USVI, and Haiti was conducted. Included in the evaluation were reviews of healthcare providers, patients, stakeholders, and community representative results, research and assessment procedures, educational outcomes, and cost-effective measurements.

Research incorporation benchmarks: Scientific examinations and analytic editorials were examined for incorporation based on the benchmarks delineated below.

Applicants: Included healthcare professionals, patients, and community populations using healthcare services to prevent the spread of COVID-19 in Africa, the USVI, and Haiti.

Interventions: Studies exploring any impact and prevention strategies related to the targeted areas identified by this book, were included in the evaluation.

Results: Study results were incorporated if they evaluated COVID-19 exposure consequences related to the healthcare services of developing countries, quality of healthcare, research, education of the population, and safety of healthcare providers as mentioned by the World Health Organization (WHO) and the U.S. Centers for Disease Control and Prevention (CDC) resource guidelines.

Date: Publication of research editorials and articles: Editorials and articles deemed valid for review, consideration, and inclusion in the book were confined to research available from January 1990 to the present.

Language: Research and articles included those available in English only; however, studies written in other languages were consulted.

Research prohibition benchmarks: Research and articles in which the impact of COVID-19 was not related to developing countries, public health improvement, and access to quality healthcare services were rejected.

Literature examination approach: The following research systems, databases, and online platforms were used to locate and identify articles within the timeline of January 1990 to the present: The Medical Literature Analysis and Retrieval System Online (MEDLINE), the WHO and CDC Database indices including African Index Medicus (AIM), Latin American and Caribbean Health Sciences (LILACS) produced by the Pan American Health Organization (PAHO) Institutional Memory Database; and the WHO Library Database (WHOLIS) using the WHO Global Health Library platform.[7]

Search Terms: The following search terms were used to focus on the scope of research for evaluation: COVID-19, the impact of COVID-19, close contact, SARS, impact of social distancing, the impact of wearing marks, African countries, the U.S. Virgin Islands, and Haiti. The literature examination also included references from retrieved reports, articles, and unofficial reports.

Choice of studies: Data retrieved from published and restricted research and articles were assessed to uncover those to be merged into the assessment. However, those which were determined not to satisfy the criteria set for inclusion in the evaluation were rejected. Review outcomes included 500 articles. Based on the criteria delineated above, 150 of these were identified not significant and therefore omitted from the evaluation. The final sum of editorials and articles considered was 350. A total of 277 were finally used as references for this work.

Research prohibition benchmarks: The evaluation rejected research and articles in which the primary aim of COVID-19 use was not related to public health prevention and access to quality healthcare services.

Variety of Coronaviruses

Coronaviridae is the name given to groups of corona viruses with the subgroups, Letovirinae and Coronavirinae. The latter has four categories, Alphacoronavirus, Betacoronavirus, Gammacoronivirus, and Deltacoronavirus; these include seven coronaviruses that can infect human beings **(Table 1).** Coronaviruses can also infect non-human mammals, **(Table 2),** and they can be carried by birds **(Table 3)** or infect them, and they can be carried by bats **(Table 4).**[8] All four types of coronaviruses are responsible for certain gastroenteric or respiratory diseases in humans and animals (**Table 5**).

Table 1. Taxonomy of coronaviruses that can cause disease in human beings.

Genus	Varieties causing human disease
Alphacoronaviruses	Human coronavirus 229E (HCoV-229E)
Betacoronaviruses	• Human coronavirus HKU1 • Human coronavirus NL63 (HCoV-NL63, New Haven coronavirus) • Human coronavirus OC43 (HCoV-OC43) • Middle East respiratory syndrome-related coronavirus (MERS-CoV or HCoV-EMC: the cause of MERS) • Severe acute respiratory syndrome coronavirus (SARS-CoV-1, the cause of SARS) • Severe acute respiratory syndrome coronavirus 2 (SARS-CoV-2 or 2019-nCoV, the cause of COVID-19)

Retrieved from Centre for Evidence Based Medecine, Nuffield Department of Primary Care Health Sciences University of Oxford; https://www.cebm.net/COVID-19/coronaviruses-a-general-introduction.

Table 2. Some non-human mammals that can be infected by coronaviruses

Animal	Variety of coronavirus
Cattle	Bovine coronavirus (BCV)—severe enteritis in calves
Cats	Feline coronavirus (FCoV)—mild enteritis in cats and severe feline infectious peritonitis
Dogs	Canine coronaviruses (CCoV)—enteritis and respiratory diseases
Ferrets	Ferret enteric coronavirus—epizootic catarrhal enteritis; Ferret systemic coronavirus—a syndrome similar to feline infectious peritonitis
Hedgehogs	Hedgehog coronavirus 1
Mink	Mink coronavirus 1
Pigs	Porcine coronavirus HKU15—gastroenteritis; Porcine epidemic diarrhea virus (PED or PEDV)
Rabbits	Rabbit enteric coronavirus—acute gastrointestinal disease and diarrhea in young European rabbits
Rats	Lucheng Rn rat coronavirus
Whales	Beluga whale coronavirus SW1

Retrieved from Centre for Evidence Based Medecine, Nuffield Department of Primary Care Health Sciences University of Oxford; https://www.cebm.net/COVID-19/coronaviruses-a-general-introduction.

Table 3. Birds that can carry or be infected by gammacoronaviruses and deltacoronaviruses

Domestic fowl: Infectious bronchitis virus (IBV)—avian infectious bronchitis
Bulbul coronavirus HKU11
Common moorhen coronavirus HKU21
Munia coronavirus HKU13
Night heron coronavirus HKU19
Turkey coronavirus (TCV)—enteritis
White-eye coronavirus HKU16
Wigeon coronavirus HKU20

Retrieved from Centre for Evidence Based Medicine, Nuffield Department of Primary Care Health Sciences University of Oxford; https://www.cebm.net/COVID-19/coronaviruses-a-general-introduction.

Table 4: Some coronaviruses carried by bats

Bat Hp-betacoronavirus Zhejiang2013
Colacovirus bat coronavirus CDPHE15
Decacovirus bat coronavirus HKU10
Miniopterus bat coronaviruses 1 and HKU8
Pipistrellus bat coronavirus HKU5
Rhinolophus bat coronavirus HKU2
Rhinolophus ferrumequinum bat coronavirus HuB-2013
Rousettus bat coronaviruses GCCDC1 and HKU
Scotophilus bat coronavirus 512
Tylonycteris bat coronavirus HKU4

Retrieved from Centre for Evidence Based Medicine, Nuffield Department of Primary Care Health Sciences University of Oxford; https://www.cebm.net/covid-19/coronaviruses-a-general-introduction.

Table 5: Diseases caused by coronaviruses

DISEASE	CORONAVIRUS TYPE
Canine coronavirus	Alpha-Coronaviruses
Feline infectious peritonitis virus	
Transmissible gastroenteritis virus	
Human Coronavirus 229E	
Human coronavirus NL63	
Porcine epidemic diarrhea virus	
Porcine deltacoronavirus	Delta-Coronaviruses
Avian infectious bronchitis virus	Gamma-Coronaviruses
MERS coronavirus	Beta-Coronaviruses
SARS coronavirus 1 (Severe Respiratory Disease)	
SARS coronavirus 2 (COVID-19)	
Human coronavirus HKU1	
Bovine coronavirus	
Human coronavirus OC43	

Retrieved from https://www.vetline.de/sites/default/files/2021-03/Fig2-relationship-corona-virus.jpg

The History of COVID-19

The origin of how the novel coronavirus (COVID-19) surfaced in Wuhan, China, continues to be the source of argument, speculation, and misinformation between China and the rest of the world. The epidemic was initially said to have begun by being spread by bats to a human being, through unhygienic marketplaces. However, several researchers do not dismiss the unfortunate accident at a research laboratory in Wuhan, China, which is believed to have possibly dispersed the deadly bat virus that had been gathered for scientific research. However, researchers have discovered, via genetic sequencing, that although it was a bat virus, the bats were not marketed at the seafood market, though several markets could have had commercialized animals that interacted with bats.

While the primary and exact cause of COVID-19 remains undetermined, a published article claims that "the focus on the origins of COVID-19 has recently turned to the possibility of a lab leak, but a zoonotic spillover is still highly likely, both for the novel coronavirus and for any future pandemic-causing pathogens."[9] Rumors were floated that the virus was created by human effort. However, the Office of National Intelligence shared the scientific community's unanimous belief that " the COVID-19 virus was not manmade or genetically modified."[10] There is also a contested hypothesis that the virus is the result of an unintended laboratory accident wherein bat coronavirus was released.[11 -13]

It is significant to highlight that during the 2003 SARS pandemic, which also originated in China, the Chinese authorities did not cooperate with the World Health Organization (WHO) in their efforts to investigate and ascertain the cause and origin of that virus. In fact, China did not volunteer information about the virus for several months; some sources say it was as long as four months. Because of this lack of cooperation, changes and reforms were requested to the International Health Regulations which regulate how countries are compelled to cope with public health disasters by imposing more stringent guidelines related to outbreak reporting.

Unfortunately, when COVID-19 began, Chinese authorities did not take into consideration their previous experiences regarding the 2003 SARS epidemic. Today, there remain challenging queries as to the roots of SARS-CoV-2, the virus that triggers COVID-19, which is now a pandemic affecting every nation on earth.

Severe Acute Respiratory Syndrome -SARS, was a transmissible and deadly respiratory disease that is said to have been caused by a coronavirus researchers called SARS-associated coronavirus (SARS-CoV). SARS-CoV is linked to SARS-CoV-2, the virus that triggers COVID-19 disease. However, there is no evidence of new occurrences of SARS having emerged since 2004.

It may take years to discover a virus in animals matching SARS-CoV-2. In the intervening time, it is vital that scientific researchers and health professionals reflect on the impending risks of other viruses and begin planning for the next outbreak. The major key to this will be working together with Chinese authorities, and the branch of the Chinese Centers for Disease Control and Prevention (China CDC). Further exploring other animal varieties and species of bats around the city of Wuhan and other parts of China, to find out what diseases and viruses they carry and transmit will be vital as this information can assist scientists in figuring out this puzzle.

Transmission and Spread

Seven types of coronaviruses can infect humans. Four are prevalent, and many people will suffer at least one of them during their lifetime.

Three of the other coronaviruses cause:

- Severe Acute Respiratory Syndrome (SARS)
- Middle East Respiratory Syndrome (MERS)
- COVID-19

These three significant and latest coronaviruses all surfaced since 2002 and have proven to be more life-threatening than other coronaviruses.[14-17] Severe acute respiratory syndrome (SARS), a virus-related upper respiratory tract infection, including the common cold, was identified as a global threat in March 2003, after first appearing in Southern China in November 2002.[18]

Researchers consider the principal way coronaviruses, such as

SARS-CoV, propagate is through close person-to-person contact with transmission believed to be via respiratory droplets (droplet spread, also called aerosol spread) produced when an infected person coughs or sneezes.

Droplet spread (>5 µm diameter, traveling <1 m) may infiltrate the mucosa of the nose or mouth - where droplet nuclei (≤5 µm diameter, which can travel >1 m) are inhaled by vulnerable persons; or may enter the eyes or upper respiratory tract via 'airborne transmission.' Droplets expelled via cough or sneeze can be propelled up to 3 feet through the air.[19-22] The viruses may remain airborne for longer duration than believed, or travel via routes not yet known by researchers.

Methods of transmitting the virus may involve:

- hugging and kissing
- sharing utensils for eating and drinking
- talking to others within a distance of 3 feet
- touching someone

If droplets from an infected individual land on an object such as a door handle or a telephone, someone else can pick up the virus if they touch these objects.[23] Several research papers show that SARS-CoV, MERS-CoV, and influenza virus might survive on a dry surface for a prolonged period, sometimes for many months. Factors influencing the survival of these viruses on surfaces include strain variation, titre, surface type, suspension medium, mode of deposition, temperature and relative humidity, and the method used to determine the viability of the virus.[24-27] Direct and indirect contact spreading is a recognized transmission path for many respiratory and gastrointestinal infections, including rhinovirus, respiratory syncytial virus, norovirus, and rotavirus.[28-32] Also, the infections are transmissible when an individual's symptoms are at their peak; however, it is likely for someone without symptoms (asymptomatic) to transmit the virus. The Centers for Disease Control and Prevention is still studying how the COVID -19 virus transmits and the seriousness of the sickness it triggers. It is essential to understand that COVID-19 is a novel infection, and studies are still in progress.

What Does "Close Contact" Imply?

In the case of COVID-19, the CDC defines *close contact* as "anyone who was within 6 feet of an infected person for at least 15 minutes starting 2 days before the onset (or, for asymptomatic patients, 2 days before positive specimen collection) of symptoms until the time the patient is isolated."[33] This is different from the definition of close contact for SARS which is defined as having cared for or lived with an individual recognized to have SARS or having a high probability of direct contact with respiratory discharges and/or body fluids of a person understood to be infected with SARS.

Examples of close contact include kissing, sharing eating or drinking utensils, close conversation (within 3 feet), physical examination, and any other direct physical contact between people. Close contact does not involve events such as walking by an individual or being seated across from someone in a waiting area or office.

In some situations, venues, and/or types of congregate settings, close contacts need additional attention and guidance on how to avoid or minimize such contact when the possibility for lesser proximity may be compromised.

How SARS-associated Coronavirus (SARS-CoV) is Caused

SARS was a zoonotic disease, suggesting it was of animal derivation but passed on to humans. According to a report published by the United Nations Environment Programme (UNEP) and the International Livestock Research Institute (ILRI), more than 60 per cent of known infectious diseases in humans, and 75% of all emerging infectious diseases are zoonotic, meaning that they come from animals.[34-35] Other scientific reports suggest that more than 6 out of every 10 known infectious diseases in humans are spread from animals, and 3 out of every 4 new or emerging infectious diseases affecting humans comes from animals.[36-37]

According to the CDC, a small number of pets worldwide, including cats and dogs, have been described to be infected with the virus that causes COVID-19, mainly after close contact with persons who have contracted the virus. However, based on information available to date, the risk of animals spreading COVID-19 to humans is still considered low. Nevertheless, the virus that causes COVID-19, SARS-CoV-2, can be spread from people to animals in some situations, mostly via contact.[38] It is another point of fact there is research showing some animals can carry a virus without being ill since their bodies are habituated to the virus, suggesting they are invulnerable.

Is COVID-19 More Dangerous than Other Viruses?

Researchers, worldwide, are battling to comprehend COVID-19, the new coronavirus that continues to infect more than 190,680,009 people globally and as of Tuesday, July 13, 2021, had caused the deaths of 4,065,496 people.[39]

Although there are many viruses in the identical category of coronavirus as COVID-19, certain of its characteristics, including its communicability, remains puzzling to scientists.

A recently published article from Jasper Hamill, a Science & Technology journalist based in London UK, revealed that Chinese researchers acknowledge the new coronavirus (COVID-19) has an 'HIV-like' mutation which helps it bind with human cells at a terrifyingly effective rate. Another study from researcher, Lu Lu, from Fudan University in Shanghai, and Jang Shibo, from the New York Blood Centre, confirmed the COVID-19 virus could attack immune systems like HIV does by targeting protective cells.[40-42] Researchers from Nankai University in Tianjin, China made available an abstract of their research wherein they state that "Because of this mutation, the packing mechanism of the 2019-nCoV may be changed and therefore be more similar to those of MHV, HIV, Ebola virus (EBoV) and some avian influenza viruses."[43-44] The abstract was previously viewable on the Chinese website Chinaxiv.org, and was also reported by the South China Morning Post which further shares that the research also implies that COVID-19's capacity to attach to cells is as much as 1,000 times greater than SARS.[45]

Both SARS and the novel coronavirus share almost 80 percent similar genetic composition.[46-48] However, it has been speculated that the "presence of a Furin site in the SARS-CoV-2 spike glycoprotein alters virulence and warrants further molecular, structural, and biophysical studies."[49] Studies of the mechanisms of transmission show for both MERS-CoV spike and SARS-CoV-2 the presence of "furin CS at the S1/S2 junction promotes entry into lung cells, and that the furin CS contributes to viral pathogenesis in SARS-CoV-2 animal models."[50- 51] According to a new study by Romeu, A. R. et al. (2021) "The furin is a serine protease widely expressed in human cells, which cleaves the SARS-CoV-2 spike at the interface of its two subunits. It is encoded by a gene on chromosome 15."[52-53] The study adds that "Furin acts on substrates with single or paired basic residues during the processing of proteins within cells. Such a polybasic furin cleavage site is found in various proteins from many viruses, including Betacoronavirus, Embecoviruses, and the Merbecovirus. However, within the betacoronaviruses of the sarbecovirus lineage B, this type of site is unique to SARS-CoV-2."

That furin is the protease responsible for both proteolytic

cleavages of HIV and SARS-CoV-2 is corroborated in the work of Hallenberger, Bosch, et al (1992), wherein they state "Furin is one protease responsible for the proteolytic cleavage of HIV envelope polyprotein precursor gp160 to gp120 and gp41 before viral assembly."[54] It has been further shown that "examination of the protein sequence of the Spike glycoprotein of SARS-CoV-2 reveals a furin cleavage sequence (PRRARS|V)."[55]

As stated earlier, SARS-CoV-2 causes COVID-19, and it is presumed that the abundance of furin proteases in the respiratory tract, and the cleaving of the SARS-CoV-2 Spike glycoprotein "upon exit from epithelial cells" can efficiently infect other cells. In contrast, the highly related bat CoV RaTG-13 does not have the furin cleavage site."[56]

Although related to severe acute respiratory syndrome (SARS) and Middle East respiratory syndrome (MERS), COVID-19 reveals some peculiar pathogenetic, epidemiological and clinical characteristics which, as yet, are not entirely known.

It is reported by the National Institutes of Health that COVID-19 can spread more easily in a community setting than its cousins, MERS and SARS, both of which are more frequently contracted in nosocomial (hospital or treatment) settings."[57]

Most cases of COVID-19 are not severe; however, the virus can trigger symptoms that turn out to be harsh, sometimes resulting in death. The epidemic of COVID-19 was abrupt, and this made it problematic to assess how frequently the infection became extremely critical and to provide accurate rates of death.

Symptoms of COVID-19

Signs and symptoms of coronavirus disease 2019 (COVID-19) may occur two to 14 days after infection. The period prior to experiencing symptoms and following symptoms of infection is known as the incubation period. This is considered to be the time between the likely initial contact source (wildlife or human being with presumed or established case) and the probable initial onset of symptoms such as cough, fever, fatigue, or myalgia.

Conventional signs and symptoms of COVID-19 can include:

- Fever
- Cough
- Fatigue
- Early symptoms of COVID-19 may include a loss of taste or smell.

Other symptoms can include:

- Shortness of breath or difficulty breathing
- Muscle pains
- Chills
- Sore throat
- Runny nose
- Headache
- Chest pain
- Recent loss of taste or smell

This list is not exhaustive and other less frequent symptoms such as rash, nausea, vomiting, and diarrhea have also been known to occur. Children have comparable symptoms to adults, but generally have milder sickness.

The seriousness of COVID-19 symptoms may vary from extremely mild too harsh. Some individuals may have only a few symptoms, while others may exhibit no symptoms. Still others may face exacerbated symptoms, such as aggravated shortness of breath and pneumonia within a week of the start of symptoms. Further, individuals who are elderly have a greater risk of substantial illness from COVID-19, with the risk increasing with age. Persons with existing chronic medical conditions (comorbid illnesses) may have a higher risk of significant sickness. Chronic medical conditions that raise the risk of substantial sickness from COVID-19 comprise:

- Serious heart diseases, such as heart failure, coronary artery disease or cardiomyopathy
- Chronic obstructive pulmonary disease (COPD)
- Type 2 diabetes
- Severe obesity
- Chronic kidney disease
- Sickle cell disease
- Weakened immune system from solid organ transplants
- Additional conditions that may add to the risk of severe disease, are:

- Asthma
- Liver disease
- Chronic lung diseases such as cystic fibrosis
- Brain and nervous system conditions
- Weakened immune system from bone marrow transplant, HIV, or some medications
- Type 1 diabetes
- High blood pressure

Again, this list is not exhaustive, and more underlying medical conditions may increase one's risk of serious illness from COVID-19.[58]

CHAPTER TWO

Coronavirus is Spreading and Challenging Recovery

While developed countries were recovering from the ravages caused by COVID-19, many developing nations including some African countries, the USVI, and Haiti, continued to cope with the repercussions of the disease outbreak. They struggled to protect the health and well-being of their populations while attempting to respond to the growing hygiene, unemployment, and severe economic needs.

Several published studies describe developing countries as third world nations, and include in this categorization South Asia, Africa, Central America, Latin America, Oceania, and the Middle East with shared significant hallmarks such as poverty, high population density, high mortality rate, economic inequity, and disparity of women to name a few.[59-61] The United Nations does not have a formal definition of developing countries. It does, however, continue to use the term for monitoring purposes and classifies as many as 159 countries as developing nations. Under the UN's current classification, all of Europe and Northern America along with Japan, Australia and New Zealand are classified as developed regions, and all other regions are developing countries.[62]

On a broad scale, these developing countries have poor economic power, labor markets, manufacturing, and education and may not sustain and recover from this disaster in the absence of effective developmental strategies and aide. Many of them are extremely vulnerable to these new worldwide diseases as they continue to endure significant challenges inherent, but not limited to their countries, which endanger their sustainable development. Their continual failure to access concessionary financing resources to develop and improve necessary resilience to natural and economic tremors is beyond their domestic management resulting in high debt levels and useless healthcare systems.

These unparalleled challenges worsen their critical vulnerability both to the COVID-19 outbreak and to any natural or man-made disaster that may occur, leaving these countries in a disadvantaged position. Given the limited resources available to them, challenges to respond, recover, and protect their population from this unprecedented COVID-19 outbreak are substantial and significant.

As of today, some of the most poorly funded and thinly staffed health systems and hospitals in the world are located in

Africa, the USVI and Haiti. Many healthcare providers struggle to receive relevant clinical information pertaining to COVID-19 from specialists, thereby confusing efforts to provide continuous, coordinated care.

Furthermore, the lack of investment in the existing systems creates greater challenges to the processes to limit the spread of the infection, as many of these developing countries continue not to invest in health infrastructure and social services, which are important determinants of health to win the fight against this unprecedented outbreak.

In these countries and throughout Africa, substantial portions of the population are uninsured because they cannot afford coverage or live-in countries that did not expand or have universal coverage, or they are unemployed. It also does not help that testing for COVID-19 may not be covered under existing health insurance even if a person is insured.

Existing insurance companies in most African countries have not waived co-payments, co-insurance, or deductibles for COVID-19 treatments. As a result, the people must pick up 100% of the cost of coronavirus testing, as copays or out-of-pocket fees are required to cover all health services, including COVID-19 testing. These costs restrain people from using testing sites such as drive-through testing at hospital off-site locations.

While it is encouraging to see the willingness to halt or decrease the spread of this disease, there needs to be a logical strategy behind chosen approaches so that everyone follows effective preventive measures. Unfortunately, accessing quality health services for testing and treatment has become a nationwide outcry as people cope with poor preventive services, unreasonable medical expenditures, and poor behavior from healthcare providers in both the public and private sectors. Despite some measures implemented and provided by governments, health structures, and primary care services, access to effective health services remains challenging for the majority of the population.

Although the U.S. Virgin Islands has structured and put in place safety and precautionary guidelines similar to those in mainland United States, the same cannot be said for Haiti and many African nations wherein safe recovery is trailing that of developed countries and undermining the well-being of their populations.

The State of the Pandemic in Africa

As multiple reports of COVID-19 surfaced from Wuhan, China in late December 2019, many African countries responded to counteract the appearance of potential first cases that would ultimately happen because of its strong relationship to China, a substantial trade ally and host to more than 80,000 Africans, mainly students.[63-66]

A 2020 statistical analysis report related to air-travel from China to Africa, confirmed that many African nations such as Egypt, Algeria, and South Africa, were at the highest risk of early exposure and spread of the virus into the African continent.[67]

These projections were presented in studies by Menkir, T.F., Chin, T., Hay, J.A. *et al.*(2021), wherein, based on aggregated data and regression analysis, it was estimated that the highest numbers of imported COVID -19 cases were expected for South Africa and Algeria, followed by Kenya, Zambia, and Egypt.[68-70] However, other reports, based on actual case reported numbers, show that although South Africa was the hardest hit with the virus, the other nations (in order of ranking for transmission of the virus) were Morocco, Tunisia, Egypt, and Nigeria, with Nigeria eventually taking second and third place.[71-73]

The vulnerability of the continent's nations to COVID-19 and other infectious diseases is strongly tied to persistent poverty, insufficient and poorly equipped health facilities, and infrastructure, along with vast areas of non-sanitary conditions and lack of access to clean, running water – facts which have been corroborated via numerous reports and studies.

Drawing on experiences from the 2014 Ebola virus outbreak in West Africa, many African countries supposedly knew that failure to suppress COVID-19 would endanger the health, prosperity, and security of their people.[74]

By the end of April 2020 many in Africa had instituted and were enforcing containment and preventive mitigation measures. These included ensuring the availability of hospital beds, protecting the vulnerable, mandating travel bans on most affected Asian and European countries, and instituted mandatory quarantine periods for the majority of travelers in an effort to curb a potential surge that would overburden the already broken health care systems. Further, these countries promptly centered not only on enforcing limits or complete lockdowns of their economies, schools, borders, and huge assemblies, but also minimizing COVID-19 importation and containing onward spread of the disease. These courses of action appeared to be effective with many African nations recording only minor cases of infection – in the beginning of the pandemic. Since the onset of the pandemic, Africa had experienced a slow but steady increase in numbers of active COVID-19 cases and deaths.

By 27 May 2020, the continent had reported relatively more than 100, 000 cases (118,717 to be exact), and 3,574 deaths spread across 47 countries.[75] While these numbers seemed to be relatively low compared to global figures (as the continent accounted for less than 1% of world-wide cases), the heartbreaking reality was that it was just the tip of the iceberg. The continent quickly began experiencing a surge in confirmed cases and deaths when they reopened their borders and began relaxing preventive measures. Of further impact was the fact that it was becoming apparent that the combined containment and mitigation preventive approaches were not working as well as expected with something as large and pervasive as COVID-19, especially as few countries were performing targeted mass screenings and testing.

The twelfth of July in 2020, there were 461,296 confirmed cases of COVID-19, including 8,092 deaths, for 47 countries that reported to the WHO.[76] From its initial outbreak to July 2020 the virus killed more people in African countries (11,955) than Ebola did in its deadliest outbreak from 2014 to 2016 in West Africa, according to the World Health Organization.[77]

While from the perspective of whole numbers, the African continent still accounted for just a tiny proportion of overall worldwide cases, the rapidly climbing rates of infection in many countries was of increasing alarm to health care specialists. Although they remained perplexed and challenged about the unprecedented surge in COVID-19 cases, public health specialists all agreed that ending lockdown restrictions, low testing capacity, isolated outbreaks, social distancing, and the virus catching up to poorly forgotten communities were each significant contributing factors.

The WHO revealed that greater than a third of countries in Africa were seeing a doubling of their case numbers within a month, and the "threat of COVID-19 was overwhelmingly foreclosing" the existing health systems.[78-80] The report attests that within 100 days the virus had caused 100,000 cases; but once it had a stronghold on the continent, within 18 days that number doubled to 200,000. Within 20 days, it doubled again.

Another report revealed that Egypt and South Africa had the highest numbers of cases with those in South Africa having surged in spite of the country enforcing one of the world's strictest lockdowns in late March; but the increase in cases came after restrictions were relaxed. Egypt, however, saw cases rise from mid-May 2020 with indications of a peak in new infections by early July.

As many on the African continent were not carrying out effective or at least targeted widespread screening and testing, their numbers, unfortunately, continued to increase. This led to an epidemiological curve comparable to those of nations more harshly hit by the virus, such as the United Kingdom, Spain, France, and the USA.[81] The CDC defines an epidemiological curve (epi curve) as "the progression of illnesses in an outbreak. Epi curves depict when people became ill by day, week, or month."[82]

At the writing of this book, the health care infrastructure in many African countries continued to demonstrate limited ability to manage viral case increases. Limitations were manifested by a lack of sufficient numbers of beds for treating active cases, a shortage of health care providers, and a major scarcity of proper personal protective equipment (PPE) for first-line health care providers. Bed capacity was projected to have been breached or overwhelmed and needed supplies such as ventilators, were still in short supply, as the ones on hand were not working or missing significant parts.

The continent's health care systems have been inadequately funded and sparsely staffed, despite efforts to improve these factors compared with the rest of the world. The WHO data reveal that the African continent has (on average) just 2.3 health care workers per 1000 people.[82]

The actual ratios of physicians per 1000 people varies

across the continent with it being 0.3 doctors per 1,000 people in Nigeria, 0.1 in Liberia, 0.2 in Sierra Leone and Ethiopia, 0.12 in Uganda, 4.3 for South Africa, and 2.8 for Egypt. Added to this dearth of adequate medical providers was that many of the available healthcare force during the pandemic were not properly trained to manage COVID.[83-84] Apprehension that a large-scale outbreak, on the heels of a humanitarian crisis, did not help ensure the safety of hospital locations or protect the few remaining dedicated health professionals. As testing became an increasingly important part of mitigating the spread of the disease along with providing proper and prompt care for those who tested positive, most of the population found themselves with few options for available laboratory testing sites.

When testing processes were performed, testing fees, uncertainty, and delays in getting screening results continued to cause anger and confusion. As the speeding surgence of viral outbreaks continued filling health care specialists with fear, what was yet frightening, was the propensity of the African people (old and young) to ignore or downplay the significant malaise that could result in tens of thousands of completely unnecessary deaths.

Health care specialists recognized people aged 65 and older to be the hardest hit primarily due to pre-existing health conditions. In the United States this population represents more than 80% of COVID-19 related deaths. There is every possibility this may also be true for Haiti and other countries in Africa, but due to the lack of readily available, accurate data, and in the absence of strictly monitored and reported epidemiological statistics, this is not known.

Although those below the age of 25 years account for more than sixty percent of Africa's 1.25 billion people, contrasted to about 42.0 percent worldwide, this demographic structure might not be one of the continent's best mitigating factors against COVID-19.[85-86]

The age profile of new infections in the coronavirus pandemic as it moved into late 2020 and early 2021seemed to be younger, following resurgences in countries associated with more social contact among those under 40 after the loosening of restrictions. Evidence from countries such as the United States, Israel, and Portugal, showed that people under 50 constituted a considerable percentage of patients requiring hospitalization.[87] The upsurge in cases among the under-40 population was criticized by health care specialists as "second wave behavior" as young people who saw themselves less likely to become infected, let down their guards. It has also been demonstrated that some viruses are often spread between people living in the same house. Therefore, a younger person with a milder, or even asymptotic case of coronavirus could still pass it to a parent, grandparent or other individual who may experience more severe symptom, have a more difficult time healing, or may have an even greater chance of dying from the virus.

The significant shift in the age profile of those being infected with the disease has led to concerns that more relaxed attitudes among the population, (older and young people) towards physical distancing, were substantial contributors to increases in the COVID-19 case rate. It is possible that these populations could have avoided infection, and the reality is that their choices about how they conduct their lives during this pandemic might prove to be the difference between life and death for someone else. Some public health specialists have been warning that people need to be more mindful of their actions during this pandemic for the benefit of themselves, families, friends, and others.

In Africa, the struggle against this prolific virus may already be lost given the continent's demographic structure and the tendency of the population (especially the young) to engage in unprecedented and risky behaviors regardless of the COVID-19 outbreak. Another point of consideration must be the lingering distrust of public health care which pushed both groups of the population to either treat themselves at home with herbal teas and various concoctions recommended by family and friends, or to seek treatment from "magic healers."

Another factor for consideration is that with the arrival of COVID-19 variants such as the DELTA, which is more highly transmissible than COVID-19, as persons 40 and younger constitute the largest percentage of populations worldwide that have not been vaccinated, it is possible we could see this demographic fall prey to the new variants.

Many Africans have shown a continued disbelief in the existence of COVID-19 as they are encumbered with greater worries regarding their daily lives. These attitudes have created barriers to people adopting and fully practicing effective preventive measures and instead, they engage in behaviors known for high transmissibility of disease such as socializing in bars and nightclubs, not social distancing, and not wearing properly required masks. Such actions help the virus to proliferate at a faster pace within communities.

The current living conditions for many Africans arose out of discriminatory policies in place over decades, as governments across the continent continued to not provide fair housing systems, a practice that kept (and still keeps) most of the poor from living decently.

The systematic denial of housing and associated services has been limiting the population's prospects and ability to acquire decent jobs and education. In turn, this has led to an over-representation of people in poverty and those working menial labor jobs, two factors preventing many from staying at home during the pandemic.

It is more challenging for people to practice social distancing in these poor communities, as residents live in small apartments or houses with a sizable number of other relatives, friends, or just guests. In these circumstances, it is less probable that the population endorsed public lockdown measures to prevent the spread of the coronavirus would be obeyed, as supportive financial measures were not implemented in most of the countries to support the population as it struggled. Viewing the transmission of disease from a socio-economic and historical perspective, the increases in virus cases makes a lot more sense as people found it necessary to continue working or finding other means of supporting and supplying needs for their families. Thus, compliance with restrictive prevention measures was not a feasible option for most citizens. Overcoming these systemic shortfalls, which lead to health inequalities that are exceptionally vivid with the COVID-19 pandemic, is essential.

The Pandemic in the US Virgin Islands (USVI)

While the COVID-19 outbreak continued unprecedented growth in many African countries, the U.S. Virgin Islands was also facing a sharp increase in confirmed cases and new rises in the number of deaths, as the territory began relaxing lockdown restrictions.

The USVI is a territory of the United States. It covers an estimated area of 346 square miles, with a population of over 104,456 people living mainly on three islands: St. Croix, St. Thomas, and St. John, according to the 2010 U.S. Census bureau.[88]

As the virus brushed across the globe, health care specialists warned of a probable dire effect on countries throughout the Caribbean which were, at the same time, trying to recover from unprecedented hurricane disasters, which left fragile economies, weak healthcare infrastructure, and thousands of people suffering. As other damaged territories economies, including Puerto Rico's, have shown substantial signs of improvement after the devastation of hurricanes Irma and Maria two years ago, the USVI economy remains hindered in a profound plunge, according to several published reports including the World Bank annual review.[89-91]

While Puerto Rico's economy is relatively diversified with some substantial industries involved in manufacturing and business services to name just a few; the Virgin Islands primary economic drivers accounting for most of its GDP and employment are tourism, trade, other services, and rum production. A 2020 analysis revealed the islands receive, on average, between 2.5 and 3 million tourists via the cruise ship industry. The same report informs that regarding recovery from the hurricanes, rebuilding continues but actual full recovery may not be achieved for some years. Effects of the hurricanes upon the healthcare systems and infrastructure remain visible and they are receiving slow remediation as gaps remain, leading to further inequities and disparities in care and reduced serviceability.[92]

The territory's hospitals on St. Croix, St. John, and St. Thomas continue to cope with substantial infrastructure damage and reductions in serviceability. Both major hospitals, Schneider Regional Medical Center on St. Thomas, and Governor Juan F. Luis Hospital on St. Croix, along with some urgent care centers, clinics, and health department facilities suffered destruction that continues to limit the services they are offering to the population.[93-94]

After experiences with two back-to-back hurricanes and their impacts on the health systems, USVI authorities knew that failure to contain COVID-19 would compromise the fragile health, prosperity, and recovery of the population. By the end of March 2020, the territory had taken significant combined containment and public health measures. Among these were: social distancing and restrictions on nonessential activities, ensuring the availability of hospital beds, protecting the vulnerable, imposing travel bans, closing schools and borders, stopping huge assemblies, and instituting mandatory quarantine periods for most travelers in an effort to curb a potential surge that would strain the already weak healthcare systems.[95] The territory also reinforced essential public health messaging such as symptom-monitoring, infection prevention and ways to avoid disease spread throughout the islands.[96] From an economic policy standpoint, the territory allocated considerable fiscal resources, extended unemployment insurance benefits, employment subsidies, temporary tax breaks and deferrals, and credit guarantees.[97] These lines of action emerged as effective, although the territory documented and reported minor cases of COVID-19 infections during that period.

In the early phases of the pandemic the islands seemed to have dodged the brunt of COVID-19, even as the worldwide outbreak besieged medical centers in neighboring islands, the U.S.A, and Western Europe. While the few reported cases appeared to be lower compared to the crushing global numbers, the disheartening realism was that it was just the calm before the storm as the U.S. Virgin Islands would soon undergo a surge in cases as they reopened and relaxed. As the pandemic raged on, the territory discovered that their combined containment and mitigation efforts were not working with something as large and complex as the virus. By 14 July 2020, there had been an increase of 217 in confirmed positive cases including 6 deaths, reported to the WHO's Dashboard.[98-99]

Compared to other territories or countries, the U.S. Virgin Islands were still only accounting for an infinitesimal fraction of total global cases; however, the increases in rates of confirmed cases and deaths were of rising alarm to government and health professionals. It was agreed that the factors of easing restrictions and not enforcing social distancing as businesses reopened could each have a considerable role in promoting disease.

Amid this concern, the CDC published a study cautioning that demographics of young and old in the U.S. and its territories were still more likely to get infected if they continued to disregard mandates and protocols enacted for their protection and to help prevent further deaths. Due to their evident vulnerability, the CDC data validated the belief that since the beginning of the pandemic, persons over 65 experienced the greatest health impacts from the virus and constituted over 80 percent of COVID-19 associated deaths worldwide; younger people, were shown also to be at higher risk.[100-102] Not abiding by the health department's guidance, the population (both old and young people) increased their chances of exposure and thereby, the chances of acquiring the virus.

St. Croix is the largest of the four islands that comprise the

USVI (St. Thomas, Water Island and St. John are the other three). At 84 square miles, St. Croix is about three times the size of St. Thomas; however, it has about the same population (over 50,601 according to the 2010 United States Census). St. John and Water Island are tiny in comparison.[103-105]

An oil refinery that was shut down some years ago for EPA violations is located on the island of St. Croix. It re-opened and set up a "man camp" where workers from off-island live in congested quarters. When the pandemic was declared, the Limetree Bay Management of the "man camp" did not tighten requirements, or track the movement of refinery workers, nor did it conduct tests of its employees on rotation at the refinery, leading the camp to become a potential COVID-19 cluster.[106-107]

Flattening the progression of the pandemic would require control of the human factors that are so critical to curbing the risk for exposure among the population. Unfortunately, well-meaning preventive measures fail because assumptions are made without full understanding of why people's behaviors exist and persist.

The Status of the Pandemic in Haiti

Applying its experience from other disasters, Haiti's government, on 16th of March 2020, proclaimed a two-week suspension of flights from Europe, Canada, the Dominican Republic, and Latin America.[108] The government also closed schools and most factories and urged the population to embrace social distancing and restrictions on unnecessary activities.[109] The island nation appeared to be successful in its efforts to thwart the disease taking the lives of so many around the globe, until March 19th 2020 when the first two cases were confirmed to have arrived in Port-au-Prince, Haiti.[110]

With only two cases, Haiti made the decision to lift restrictions, reopening textile factories, (which account for 90 percent of the country's exports), loosening mandates on mask wearing, participation in unnecessary activities, and even relaxed social distancing.[111] In this way, the Haitian government exposed the lives of its most vulnerable people to the deadly virus.

On 4 June 2020, Doctors Without Borders (Médecins Sans Frontières) voiced serious concerns "that because of the easing of restrictions of preventive measures, the COVID-19 cases in Haiti have been increasing fast in less than one month from 100 cases to more than 2,600 cases and 50 deaths." It was further noted that the existing healthcare capacity could not support the surge in cases and deaths.[112] By 16 July 2020, an increase of 6,831 confirmed positive cases, including 143 deaths, had been reported to the WHO's Dashboard.

The health care infrastructure in Haiti has shown limited capacity to cope with case increases, including having insufficient numbers of beds for treating COVID-19 patients, a shortage of healthcare providers, and a major scarcity of proper personal protective equipment (PPE) for healthcare workers and providers. Before the pandemic hit the small island nation there were expressed concerns about the safety of hospitals chosen for treatment of coronavirus patients and the ability to protect community health providers given the decimated state of health infrastructure and inadequate resources.

Testing, too, became an important challenge in efforts to mitigate the spread of the disease as the Haitian people found themselves with only two laboratories in the entire country able to process COVID-19 tests, including rapid diagnostic tests (RDTs). Added to this scenario was that once testing was performed, it was followed by uncertainty, delay, and confusion regarding the screening results, causing anger in the population. It was reported that although the Public Health Ministry allowed only PCR tests, it usually took ten days to get results to patients, while a private Med Lab center using the fluorescent immunoassay (FIA) test was able to contain the cost at 6,250 gourdes ($57.00) and give same day results.[113] The Public Health Ministry and Population agency fought back claiming that the private Med Lab could not administer the FIA test, and that it was too expensive for the population already experiencing economic distress and declared only PCR testing would be allowed.

The 2019 revision of the World Population Prospects revealed that the total population of Haiti in 2018 was 11,123,178, compared to only 3,221,000 in 1950.[114] The proportion of children below the age of 15 in 2010 was 36.2%; the population between the ages of 15 and 65 accounted for 59.7%, while those 65 and older constituted only 4.5% of the total population. This population graph is in stark contrast to Haiti's population in 2019 wherein those 0-14 account for 33%; 15-64 were 62%, and 65 and older 5%. Add to this that 24.7 percent of the population lives in extreme poverty which equates to a wage of less than $1.25 per day, and more than 59 percent live on less than $2.00 per day.[115-117] These data are significant in the COVID-19 pandemic environment because the poor are less likely to have access to quality health care and tend to live in poorly ventilated, crowded housing wherein disease can spread more easily.

Amid the pandemic, the tiny island nation has been trying to survive many shock waves, including civil unrest, hurricanes, floods, resurgence of preventable communicable diseases (primarily TB- the highest incidence in the western hemisphere and cholera), death, staggering unemployment, and lack of quality health care. Added to the country's woes, this pandemic has proven to be a complex adversary as Haiti faces significant challenges in its efforts to mitigate and contain the virus. Lack of faith in and disbelief of the public healthcare system, and mistrust of government and public health authorities, and not sensing any initial sincerity about enforcing the health department's guidance, all these coalesced to create an environment ripe for disease proliferation. Stories have circulated that so distrustful is the general populous, that many have resorted to home remedies such as herbal teas as treatment. These factors undermine any hope of the compliance with the mandated measures.

Daily survival is a primary barrier to enforcement of proven prevention measures. Gross poverty causes people to seek employment in nefarious and often dangerous conditions and professions, many of which put people in contact with those who have communicable and sexually transmitted diseases and COVID-19. Even if they believed authorities, the impetus to provide for daily survival outweighs any fear of contracting diseases.

Poor infrastructure, compromised sanitation systems and inadequate access to clean water continue to be massive deterrents to disease mitigation and containment, creating horrific disparate conditions. Only half of the population in the capital city of Port-au-Prince and its surrounding areas have access to the public water network, and only half of the rural populous has access to pipes and other improved water infrastructure and sources.

With most Haitians earning their income through informal work such as fishing, direct services, or street vending, necessary public health measures including social distancing and restrictions on nonessential activities, were not only difficult to enforce, but strict enforcement would ruin the fragile household earnings of already brutally impoverished families.

Stories, misinformation, and cultural beliefs did not help. Haitian attitudes about COVID-19 risk were associated with tribal culture and how people see the world in spite of prevailing facts. One of the more widely circulated conspiracy theories about COVID-19, is that it is a hoax (believed by 60% of the population interrogated). Another is that because the virus emerged in China, it could not reach Haiti (a claim believed by as much as half the population) because of the distance and that somehow the virus could be killed by the large oceans. This may appear counterintuitive because better-educated Haitians are more likely to be mindful of the scientific information related to the virus. However, in the judgment of the poor and the suffering, COVID-19 is not a scientific fact, it is a political or man-made issue.[118-121]

As COVID-19 is an infectious disease that is highly dependent on human hosts for transmission, the more people act as normal socializing beings, the greater the chances the virus has to replicate and spread. Unfortunately, the massive distrust of government has caused most Haitians to lack the motivation to acquiesce and change their behaviors - even for the benefit of mitigating disease spread among their own homes and communities. Coupled with elements of poverty and deteriorating living conditions, compliance to practicing positive behaviors could have been the turning point between life and death for many.

An economic and social byproduct of all this has been the continual depreciation of the gourde, (Haitian currency), a steady rise in food prices, and new restrictions on movement and disruption of economic activities, causing the most vulnerable Haitians to be pushed deeper into poverty.

CHAPTER THREE

The Impact of Delusion and Denial

People Living as if There Were No Pandemic

As COVID-19 cases rose, people in Africa and Haiti flouted health mandates and rules with parties, beach days, vacations, work, and even assuming the coronavirus outbreak never occurred and if it did, it would just blow away.

In the USVI, the government began addressing COVID as early as February 2020, establishing a Coronavirus (COVID-19) Task Force to lead the charge against the outbreak. By March 23, a stay-at-home order was issued mandating all islanders, with the exception of essential workers, remain at home. All non-essential government operations were shut down, the Bureau of Tourism shut its doors, and evictions and rent collections were suspended. It would appear that the Island was taking serious and definitive measures to stem what was proving to be a deadly virus. However, beaches – a mainstay of many islanders and visitors – remained open until April 6; and when finally shut down, were closed only through April 20 – a mere two weeks. [122] Thus, although people were home, many were congregating on the beaches, thereby, helping to spread the virus.

In conversations with friends and various people in official capacities throughout the islands, it was shared that many people did not heed the restrictions or practice the preventive measures. Some claimed the virus was not real, or that because of their not being elderly, it would not affect them. Still, others had a lassaiz faire attitude believing "if I'm going to get it, I'm going to get it no matter what."

In Haiti, the crisis of the COVID-19 pandemic has had even greater ramifications. A struggling health infrastructure with the capacity to treat only "a few hundred patients at a time" could not handle increases in patient volume stemming from impacts of the virus. In fact, according to 2019 studies conducted by the Research and Education Consortium for Acute Care in Haiti (REACH) the island nation of greater than 11 million was estimated to have 124 ICU beds and 64 ventilators. This reality is further compounded by the fact that the government does not provide sufficient funding for its national response planning.[123-124]

In speaking with contacts residing in Haiti, it was revealed that people were not taking the risk of getting the virus seriously despite rises in case numbers and deaths. It was not helpful that the media continued to report that overall Haiti had not experienced predicted death tolls that were projected due to the weakened infrastructure, poor health care, and other problems that are ripe conditions for a contagious disease to proliferate.

In a country where weather is warm and poverty is rampant, people were seen walking the streets, going to markets, and conducting other activities with carelessness in sizeable crowds. Strict directives were posted, along with photos and videos, on social media showing citizens acting as if life were normal and all the talk about risks were exaggerated. Social distancing was useless as people walked shoulder-to-shoulder on city streets without wearing face masks or appropriate cloth coverings, exposing themselves and others to possible virus particulate matter.

It has been said that many believed the virus was under control and they could therefore gather in bars, restaurants, nightclubs, and markets. Alongside that belief was the claim that the seriousness of the virus had been downplayed publicly and was further minimized by the hysteria surrounding it. Even most businesses made public their willingness to remain open despite government and public health restrictions. Many argued that city mandates were unlawful. Employees, fearful of losing already meager wages, supported business owners' refusals to comply with pandemic guidance. Thus, many businesses did not close, and this helped the pandemic spread.

The environment created by this blatant ignoring of public health mandates put the lives and safety of the elderly, the disabled, and others at high risk for the virus, at jeopardy. Media in the United States and other Western and more developed nations spread the news that younger people were less likely to get the virus or incur serious illness if they did, causing this demographic to be even more blatant in its refusal to adhere to restrictions. Thus, this sub-group became likely spreaders of the virus as it was determined that many such persons were probably asymptomatic. This behavior, coupled with inaccurate beliefs and assumptions was a risky gamble for not only Haitians, but also in the USVI, where case numbers appeared low, but began to surge there and in the nations of Africa. Almost eight months into the pandemic, ample evidence emerged showing that the virus was deadlier than the seasonal flu, resulting in more deaths over shorter periods of time.

In recent years as societies around the globe have displayed more egocentric behaviors and approaches to public facing issues, that attitude has also become prevalent in Africa, the USVI, and Haiti. The result of this 'me attitude' is that in this pandemic people have continually disavowed adherence to the guidance of top national and international health entities (the CDC, the NIH, and the WHO) with the cry that these infringe upon their personal freedoms. Little to no consideration is given that a public health disaster affects everyone and can become insidious if all do not cooperate with preventive guidance and measures.

A direct outgrowth of this egocentric predominance has been that people tend not to be as compassionate toward those who may suffer greater malaise and effects of the virus. In the United

States, this became acutely apparent when a governor commented that the elderly were willing to die rather than allow businesses to suffer because of closures due to COVID-19.[125] There seemed to be a nationwide belief that lives of the elderly were of no consequence and were being allowed to die by the thousands in nursing homes. In Italy more than 7,000 elderly died in nursing homes from COVID-19.[126,127] Unfortunately, this attitude was adopted in countries where healthcare is sketchy, poverty is the standard, and access to clean water and sanitation are sorely compromised, helping to create a breeding ground for the spread of disease.

The World Health Organization (WHO) disclosed that "although all age groups are at risk of contracting COVID-19, older people face a significant risk of developing severe illness if they contract the disease because of physiological changes that come with aging and potential underlying health conditions.[128]

The Centers for Disease Control and Protection (CDC) warned that also at high risk for serious illness were those with weakened immune systems, and "they may also remain infectious for a longer period than others with COVID-19."[129] Therefore, helping and protecting older persons and those with immunocompromised systems should have been everyone's concern and everyone's business. In short, the principle of beneficence should have prevailed as the order of the day. Ample evidence has shown that countries that were more collective and considerate of the entire population had more effective leverage in flattening the curve of COVID-19 spread because they focused on the health and well-being of everyone instead of just portions of the population.

It is not farfetched to assume that several months into stay-at-home orders most people would be at their wits' end. However, evidence has demonstrated that developed countries that followed strict recommendations such as stay-at-home orders and wearing a face mask or appropriate face cloth, alongside applying social distancing, were successful in reopening with fewer glitches. This shows that a collective understanding of the dangers of the virus and at-risk behaviors were more rational and emotionally positive approach than pretending the risk did not exist.

While it is normal to be afraid of the unknown, and the COVID-19 pandemic is filled with uncertainty, denial of the existing reality and unwillingness to face the certainty that it can lead to prolonged serious illness and death is a cruel and ill-fated coping mechanism with repercussions not only for those ignoring the orders to prevent and protect themselves but can be a death sentence to others less able to physically fight off the disease.

Denial as a National Narrative

Several months after the first cases of COVID-19 were reported, populations in Africa, the USVI, and Haiti were still struggling to adjust to life in the new pandemic environment.

By July 19 July 2020, the number of combined confirmed cases in the African continent, USVI, and Haiti had increased to more than 586,3497 including 9,609 deaths, stressing already poorly equipped health systems.[130]

In the summer of 2020, much more information about the virus, its origin, how it behaved, and the depth of illness it could cause, was well known and shared around the world. The entire globe found itself locked in a battle against the disease with some nations enforcing strict behavioral codes (The United States, some African nations, many of the Caribbean and Central American islands including Haiti, China, Italy and many more), with others deciding to rely on people's intelligence to dictate what precautions they would take (Sweden, South Korea, Turkmenistan).[131-132]

There were, within all nations, factions that refused to take the virus seriously. Denials were peppered with myths and conspiracy theories touting it was a political ploy, it was a rumor, a myth, it was created using computers and even that the danger had been exaggerated by a cabal of shady individuals out to recreate a new one-world government and economy. A myriad of other unsubstantiated theories prevailed even when loved ones were diagnosed with the disease and some died. These untruths were spread via the social media and conservative news outlets. It seemed there was a suspension of reality, as most people believed all they had to do was just imagine the virus was fictive and they could return to living their lives as usual.

Another denial and delusion that spread through countries, especially in Africa and Haiti, was the assertion that the populations of these areas would "catch nothing," because they may already have developed antibodies to stop the virus's spread because of being born in tropical countries.[133]

It was difficult to dispel the myths, lies, and blatant misinformation because some of the sources were deemed credible. The constant irregularity of messaging within public health and government agencies and among specialists contributed to population uncertainty, which was exacerbated by the creation of confusion in how and where the population was to receive news and information. For many, especially young groups for whom the primary source of news is clickbait's or soundbites, it was easy to get incorrect and/or inaccurate messages.

Not discussed, but possibly another underlying component in the chain of steadfast denial, was the pride factor. Pride kept people from acknowledging their shortcomings in the face of a fatal disease. All these beliefs coalesced, causing the COVID-19 pandemic to remain a stunning, skeptical, and surreal phenomenon for most humans.

Something else to consider along with denial is that people's refusal to cover their nose and mouth was perhaps vanity-driven and politically underscored. Whether or not to wear a face mask has grown into a clash of cultures among the compliant and others who ardently counterattack the commands and recommendations of government and public health specialists as a matter of principle to preserve individual rights and believed constitutional freedoms. Some in authority are boldly among those who continued to send signals through their words and actions that COVID-19 was a dupery which no longer held a severe risk and therefore, people could resume business as normal without compliance to public health mandates and recommendations.

Another segment of the population that adamantly ignored the precautions were ardent church goers and believers in healing by faith. This group continued to attend church services en masse, spouting the belief that they were covered by the blood of Jesus Christ and their faith in Him, would prevent disease from attacking them.

This was not only the case in African countries and Haiti, but even in the United States, where many fundamentalist churches refused to adhere to scientific and medical supported evidence of COVID's contagion. Pastors and religious leaders with no education in medicine or sciences, relying on their interpretation of Holy Scripture, encouraged their congregants to forego obedience to established local and federal regulations even though the same Holy Scriptures admonish them to obey the laws of the land and those in authority over them (King James version of the Bible, Hebrews 13:16; Romans 13: 1, 2). Religious leaders gave advice about social distancing and face masks being a needless and fear-driven overreaction. It is unfortunate, but the reality is that despite the rational belief in the power of God, the certainty is that such denial does and did not protect against the deadly virus.

Today, in the face of the severity of millions of infections and hundreds of thousands of deaths, many pastors and religious leaders have apologized, backpaddled, or re-qualified their previous comments. Of course, correlation does not equal causation, but together with the narratives of denialists dying and previous studies showing that belief in medical conspiracy theories is related to lower rates of compliance with medically suggested health behaviors, these outcomes offer an unambiguous picture of how believing in and spreading medical misinformation can be fatal.

Although it is not yet clear just how broad the death gap might be among those who believed in the wisdom of closing the countries in the name of social distancing contrasted to those who did not, COVID-19 does not and did not distinguish between believers and non-believers. During a viral pandemic, neither belief nor denial is an effective juju or amulet to wash away disease compared to the need for shared acceptability of protective actions by society as a whole. Belief in misinformation has a capacity for harm, and in the case of COVID-19, that harm amounted to losing human lives.

Dr. Vivek Murthy, the U.S. Surgeon General serving in the Biden administration, in his first surgeon general's advisory release corroborated that "the "urgent threat" posed by the rise of false information around COVID-19 is one that continues to put "lives at risk" and prolong the pandemic."[134] However, getting denialists to accept the necessity for social distancing, emergency shelter-at-home orders, and other vital restrictions to curb the spread of infection is challenging as the reason for these denials appears to be part psychological and part cultural.

The American Psychological Association defines "psychological denial" as "a defense mechanism in which unpleasant thoughts, feelings, wishes, or events are ignored or excluded from conscious awareness. It may take such forms as the refusal to acknowledge the reality of a terminal illness, a financial problem, an addiction, or a partner's infidelity. Denial is an unconscious process that functions to resolve emotional conflict or reduce anxiety."[135]

Further, psychological denial is a personal problem with public ramifications when people are in a state of denial that leads to their engaging in behaviors that affect the welfare of others. One study contends that the ability to use denial is even "a normal stage of child development," and (on occasions) can be a beneficial adaptation in adulthood if it momentarily supports people to cope with unbearable emotions and opinions.[136] William S. Meyer, a renowned clinical social worker, and an associate professor of psychiatry at Duke University Medical Center, claimed that "Initially, in a time of crisis, a certain amount of denial is healthy because this gives a person time to acclimate to things that are frightening or painful."[137]

Expressed differently, denial is only beneficial when it is a momentary substitute action that assists people in recognizing a frightening, undesirable reality (such as COVID-19) and then, maybe, take action about the issue. In the case of COVID-19, denial can also be the consequence of feelings of helplessness and hopelessness which become desperate defenses against unhappiness related to the overwhelming and unclear landscape of the pandemic situation. It is essential that people get affirmation of hope to minimize denial, thereby leading to productive and healthy behaviors.

While some African nations managed comparatively well to somehow contain the pandemic with visible transmission chains in urban areas and remote and rural localities, there was also a disturbing increase in the number of asymptomatic cases, with embedded chains of transmission that remained undetectable. Although few groups of people living in those localities denied community transmission of coronavirus, it was an assertion broadly rejected by many who argued that although travel prohibitions had been established, the virus had spread among groups that engaged in very little travel or had no contact with travelers.

Meanwhile, community transmission, (which implies person-to-person spread of an infection where the source is difficult to trace), coupled with denial, had troubling repercussions. Limited healthcare resources were used to attempt tracing of transmission chains in areas with community transmission when those resources should have been committed to quarantining and treating the infected. Denying community transmission not only sent out the incorrect message at a point when every other person should have been considered, theoretically, contaminated, but also people continued to believe there was no threat in not adhering to preventive protocols for public behavior.

If there is one lesson from the worldwide response to COVID-19, it is this: The countries that have had the most success in "flattening the curve" acted at once and forcefully to suppress the virus, rather than denying or downplaying the risk it presented.

This virus has the propensity to be catastrophic but hopefully, lessons learned in this first wave will serve as a wake-up call for governments and populations, especially young people, to reevaluate their priorities and not take life's generous gifts for granted.

Finally, while the COVID-19 outbreak continues, African countries, the USVI and Haiti should take their fates into their own hands because, as truly echoed by philanthropists Bill and Melinda Gates, "Every life has equal value," and "Every person deserves the chance to live a healthy, productive life."[138-139]

The Dilemmas of Social Distancing and Face Coverings

It had been over a year into the pandemic and many African countries and the USVI finally sided with the rest of the globe in enforcing strict guidelines to suppress the pandemic's surge, while Haiti maintained its more relaxed approach.

In the beginning and at the height of the pandemic restrictive guidelines mandated that people should wear masks in public, stand 6 feet apart and remain indoors unless they were essential workers or in emergency conditions, until further notification. Although most people followed the restrictions by working remotely and foregoing travel, there were many who perceived these restrictions as an overreaction from governments and public health specialists.

Ample evidence such as social media posts and published articles coupled with our field assessments showed that large numbers of people continued to disregard public health rules despite scientific indications showing adherence would prevent and halt the transmission of COVID-19. Many defiantly ran toward the exact things public health specialists cautioned against taking advantage of discounted travel, packing into overcrowded bars or nightclubs, and standing firm attending public venues and community gatherings.

Although many of these countries have a much younger population than developed nations, (and this may have helped to reduce the spread of COVID-19 cases), millions of them suffer from HIV/AIDS, malnutrition, tuberculosis, and other respiratory infections, which could enhance their vulnerability to the virus and its impacts. At the height of the pandemic there were older persons refusing to cancel their plans, likely because of a "been there, done that" mentality of having survived other worldwide epidemics, such as HIV/AIDS and Ebola.

By November 2020, the rapid rise of COVID-19 rates had approached 14,765,256 million globally, with a combined total of 631,259 cases in Africa, the USVI, and Haiti.[140] Social distancing appeared to be among the most effective preventive measure available as it helped limit contact between infected individuals and those not infected, and if implemented could prevent millions of deaths. As long as large social congregations remained constant and long-standing, social distancing or staying 6 feet away from others continued to be challenging to implement. It was challenging to embrace such sudden recommended changes to people's daily routines, along with the open-ended possibility that the recently adopted scenario could become the new normal, at least until a vaccine was developed.

The uncertainty about when COVID-19 would end, poor access to information, and underlying beliefs influenced most people to ignore preventive measures. As risky and speculative the notion of invulnerability was, most people looked at COVID-related news and remained fearless despite the images of sick and dying patients. Those who continued resisting compliance to preventive behaviors had not reached a point where they felt enough personal risk and did not have an acute perception of altruism or beneficence that would move them to compliance in the interest of saving others irrespective of any perceived cost to their own personal freedoms. Instead, the desire to self-define one's existence regardless of how any implicit choices would affect others became the prevailing rallying cry propelling ever greater numbers of people to the side of disregarding preventive public actions. For some, it was not disregard for others, but rather the expression of frustration in response to the loss of social norms and other stressors affecting them and family - some brought about by their choice of inaction, which was itself, action.

As 2021 came into view and the promise of possible vaccines seemed more imminent, there was a perception of goal achievement as people sensed COVID-19 was over and life seemed to be returning to normal. This, however, only served to provide another false perception of protection. Assuming the curve had been flattened and the worst was behind them, there was even less desire to follow public health orders, including social distancing and wearing face masks.

The fight against COVID-19 spiraled into a political and societal battle, wherein people were emotionally and mentally exhausted. Their shared novel way of life that kept them from visiting family and friends, and going about, and what they considered, business as usual took an enormous psychological toll.

Children found themselves out of school. For parents, alternative types of childcare were difficult to arrange. School-age children and youth experienced disruption to the normal course of their lives and social and emotional development and were scarred in different ways by pressures to maintain social distancing and wear masks. Added to all this were gross economic losses, difficulties in meeting necessary expenditures such as rent and putting food on the table. It was no surprise that people were fighting against the constraints even though they were in place to protect them and their loved ones.

In Africa and Haiti, the rules were especially oppressive as many made their living as street vendors, or open-air market purveyors of goods; for these, wearing masks was not an issue, but social distancing and lockdowns were. People were accustomed to crowded, lively markets where bartering and bickering over the costs of goods was an expected occurrence performed with people arm-to-arm and face-to-face. In this new mandatory and enforced environment incomes were suddenly gone or woefully decreased.

Unpublished reports, paired with our field assessments, revealed that in Africa and Haiti most people work in these informal sectors without contracts of any kind, unaided by unemployment insurance, or benefit of continued salary if business unexpectedly ceases. An unanticipated consequence of this was that in areas where food scarcity was already problematic, losses in meager income causing increased lack of access to food. Lack of food meant greater disease propensity and overall difficulty in remaining healthy.

While African countries, the USVI, and Haiti acted to avoid large outbreaks, the prospect of enforcing a lockdown, was challenging for many people, whose daily lives were already difficult because of the significant poverty gap in which they lived. Although a virus does not differentiate between poor and rich, it is more complicated for an impoverished population to protect themselves on multiple fronts beyond just the virus.

A large share of many of these countries' urban populations live in overcrowded, informal communities in tiny one or two-bedroom houses. Although differences across these three areas are large, on average, in Haiti and Africa most households share toilets with their neighbors and their only access to clean water is from a communal tap. Therefore, expecting people residing in these household conditions not to leave their homes was more than impractical, it was unrealistic and added another layer of hardship and concern. In such instances, addressing the social-distance-conscientious objectors it should have been understood that their choice to not adhere to recommended public health mandates, despite reasonable arguments and the danger to the remaining population, was rooted in equally dire conditions that affected their ability to continue living.

Social distancing was, and remains, a social protection measure to ensure that most people across countries are not carrying the burden of slowing the disease alone. Although the enemy, (COVID-19), remained invisible and normalcy was gone, social distancing is and was not social isolation. People found ways to use technology such as FaceTime, Google Duo, Zoom, WebEx, other teleconference platforms, text messaging, and email to foster continued interactions with others and to conduct business, all while remaining safe and protected.

As the outbreak was surging worldwide there was unanimity that one of the simplest approaches to curb the transmission of the infection was to wear a face mask or appropriate cloth face covering over the nose and mouth. Within the first few months of the pandemic's surge face mask wearing went from needless for healthy people to being compulsory for everyone who ventured outdoors being urged to wear them, causing a kind of psychological whiplash as people tried to figure out what was fact and what was fiction about the pandemic.

This approach was endorsed by the WHO and the CDC. In an amended statement the WHO asserts that it "promotes and offers guidance on the use of face masks or appropriate cloth face covering in communities, home care, in health care settings, and areas which have reported cases of COVID-19."[141] Previous CDC protocol for wearing face masks asserted that, "face masks or appropriate cloth face coverings should primarily be worn by those who are sick merely to prevent the transmission of germs to others."[142]

The CDC guidelines were changed to encourage all people to use face masks or appropriate cloth face coverings in public spaces. The agency stated that along with masks, "the spread of COVID-19 can be reduced when face coverings are used along with other preventive measures, including social distancing, frequent hand-washing, and cleaning and disinfecting often touched surfaces." It was continually stated that "wearing face masks would help protect people around you, including those at higher risk of severe illness from COVID-19 and workers who often come into close contact with other people (e.g., in stores, hospital, and restaurants) from catching the virus."[143, 144] Further, the CDC clarified: "who should NOT use face masks or appropriate face clothes: children under age 2, or anyone who has trouble breathing, is unconscious, incapacitated or otherwise unable to remove the mask without assistance." The CDC added that public face masks or appropriate cloth face coverings should NOT be surgical masks or N95 respirators, as these are critical supplies which should be reserved for healthcare workers and other first responders."[145, 146]

Imposing the compulsory donning of masks or other appropriate cloths ensured that viral spread by any potential carrier was substantially diminished. Too, it underlined the concept of source control, regulating the volume of a pathogen present in the surrounding environment.

Further, face-coverings have proven to be an effective barrier between people's respiratory droplets being inadvertently shared and possibly causing infection. An added value of the ubiquitous face masks is the decreased risk that respiratory droplets will be discharged to end on surfaces or for lesser aerosolized particles to float in the air.

During the height of the disease ample evidence suggested if every person wore a face mask, droplet spreading from each individual would decrease and reduce risk, saving at least 130,000 lives over three months.[147] The more masked people in public, the less prospect for the virus to disseminate. Viral transmission via asymptomatic persons is reduced by face coverings; any other disease impact via coughing, sneezing, etc., is also diminished by the wearing of face coverings. An added societal and psychological benefit is that the wearing of a face covering may be construed as demonstration of one's concern for others.

In a cough test simulator laboratory demonstration conducted by Florida Atlantic University,[148] it was found that droplets released from a heavy cough without a mask immediately traveled 3 feet, 6 feet in 5 seconds, and 9 feet in ten seconds; in 1 minute, the droplets had traveled 12 feet and remained in the air for at least 2 minutes. A simulated light cough was also shown to immediately travel 3 feet.

Additional simulations included coughing into a hand – droplets were still dispersed from between fingers and around the outer edges of the mouth; and with a mask on, droplets escaped from the edges of the mask. In these two simulations droplets did not travel as far as in the other simulations without a mask, clearly demonstrating that wearing a mask does have prevention ability to a significantly larger degree than not wearing a face mask or covering. The wearing of a bandana as a face mask had the same effect as not wearing a mask at all as droplets immediately traveled 3.5 feet. Simulations by other universities and professional scientific laboratories gave similar, and in many cases, the exact same results.[149-152]

These simulations point to some inescapable and undeniable facts: the wearing of face masks is a better shield against the virus than not wearing one, and the social distance requirement of at least 6 feet between persons means less contact with virus particulate and aerosol droplets. Further, it was found that talking spread viral droplets even more than coughing; again, reinforcing the need and justification for social distancing and mask wearing.

[153] Evidence was also found to support the wearing of face masks as being effective in keeping economies viable and productive resulting in fewer closures of businesses.[154]

African nations, the USVI, and Haiti pride themselves on individuality. In a pandemic that required concerted endeavors to support everyone's' health and well-being, that individuality was proven to be more of a vice than a virtue. Whether or not people complied with public health mandates with ease came down to what kind of culture was preeminent: was it a highly radical 'me' culture or a 'we' culture?

For the most part, people have a predilection toward individuals making their own decisions and local government determinations hold some sway but may meet resistance. This was not the case in places where effective public health strategies were formulated and successful in hindering viral spread. In those nations people were willing to forego their personal freedoms for the benefit of the many and did not view it as a sacrifice to live out the principle of beneficence in action.

In countries where resistance to mask wearing was profound, it was not the "oh-that-mask-does not-go-with-your-clothing" type of resistance; rather, the ugliness was a cultural-political struggle as people felt personal control over areas of their lives had been taken from them.

Detractors said mask recommendations infringed upon their liberty and were a means of repression, conspiracy, and even blasphemy. Some believed that not wearing face masks made sense because they needed to have control, or at least the perception of it in order to survive and thrive as a species and as individuals. The argument stated that since they had grown to take ownership of their lives and were intrinsically social beings, COVID-19 was causing them to go against nature. It did not help that for the people of Africa and Haiti, past viral and other disease epidemics had occurred but those had not resulted in societal changes, businesses had not shut down, people had not been sequestered to their homes to alleviate the spread of disease. These differences made adapting to the pandemic behavior guidelines far more difficult, adding to the resistance to health mandates.

In places where face mask-wearing was still not an acceptable practice despite government and public health recommendations, people who wore masks were ostracized or even harassed. A sizable minority of the population - worldwide - perceived face mask-wearing as a sign of weakness revealing people were frightened. Some refusing the mask mandate purported their resistance was a sign of self-empowerment.

There were also differences in how men and women viewed masks. Our field assessments revealed that men were more willing to opt out of wearing them, believing the coverings to be "disgraceful," "a sign of vulnerability" despite data showing men were at a substantially greater risk than women of dying from COVID-19.

It would have been helpful if people had viewed the masking mandate as a preventive measure that although inconvenient, was a fact-based guideline that was apolitical, nondiscriminatory, and thoroughly grounded in science. The science and the data were very clear: wearing masks was (and is) the single best mitigation approach to suppress the spread of COVID-19. It was the strongest path to keeping people and their families safer, to keeping people out of the hospitals, and maintaining some economic viability as more businesses could remain open.

Overall, governments and public health professionals continually reminded the populations to protect not only the most vulnerable but themselves as well by avoiding the *Three C's: Closed Spaces, Crowded Places, and Close-Contact Settings* and wearing a mask in public.

Refusal to be Tested and the Importance of Testing

Even with the blatant reality of COVID-19 cases and deaths steadily rising, millions continued to refuse to be tested for the virus. If there is one lesson, the world has learned in COVID-19's outbreak it is that testing for the virus is indispensable. This fact is true for all contagious diseases, but especially for viruses such as COVID-19 that have the propensity to spread rapidly throughout a population. The capacity to identify who has the infection and who does not, offers vital information that leads to fast detection of cases, rapid therapy for those found to be positive for the virus, and urgent quarantine to avoid transmission. Early testing also facilitates identification of persons who may have been in contact with an infected individual so they too can be treated.

Worldwide, by 30 July 2020, upwards of 16,812,755 million confirmed cases of COVID-19, including 662,095 deaths, had been reported to the WHO.[155] As of early July, of Haiti's 11.26 million people only 89,917 (approximately 0.8%) had been tested for COVID-19.[156] At the height of the pandemic in 2020, less than 1 percent (actually 0.1%) of the African population had been tested.[157] By July 2021, 56,619 people on the continent had been tested; this number accounts for just 0.04% of Africa's 1.29 billion population.[158] In the same time frame as Africa and Haiti, the USVI had tested 48,881 people, constituting 47% of the island's population.[159]

The testing numbers for Haiti and Africa are significant when coupled with the fact that even public health specialists have admitted that mask wearing in Haiti, as well as the observance of preventive mandates is not something with which the population complied or took seriously. Dr. Jean "Bill" Pape, one of the top infectious disease specialists in Haiti, when interviewed, actually stated "most people do not wear masks."[160] It is also quite probable that a large percentage of Haiti's populous already had COVID-19. This is evidenced by the fact that 90 percent of those tested in the capital, Port Au Prince, tested positive, and throughout the country many reported having family members and friends who displayed symptoms of the virus, but did not seek medical care or demonstrate excessive symptoms. This general report was substantiated by Dr. Pape, who admits that "Some have all symptoms, but most have a very mild disease."[161]

Once testing began in earnest, incorrect assertions were made that increases in viral cases were due to increased testing. Ample evidence, however, revealed that the rise in cases during that time was also correlated to nations relaxing precautions, especially in rural and remote areas. In Haiti, what restrictions did exist were seldom adhered to due to economic hardship and poverty which meant people had to be out and about conducting business as usual. The is very likely true for many areas of Africa citizens rely upon informal businesses for income.

Of equally greater importance is that as of December 2020 the majority of restrictions had been lifted, meaning life as usual was resumed in the island nation, thereby allowing the virus free rein. Of course, there are also arguments that the primary reason behind Haiti's low numbers and rates of infection are due to the youth of its population wherein the average age is 23, and the virus is not known to affect the young to the degree it does those above the age of sixty.

More than anything, the data for Haiti and Africa may be taken as an implication there is no verifiable and accessible data to determine the extent of the disease's spread in the rest of the populations and what happens to the remaining 99 percent in these two areas remains a puzzle. Concerted and accountable testing would solve this data insufficiency and the gap in testing of these significantly large populations.

The World Health Organization said the best approach to defeat COVID-19 is by "testing, testing, testing", but as noted by the data, the African continent and Haiti were still testing fewer people in comparison to developed countries such as China, South Korea, the USA, Italy, and Germany according to the WHO. [162] These gaps in testing and the differing progression of the disease in each country continues, even today, to raise concerns among health professionals as to whether these countries, without increased testing, can say with certainty how COVID-19 transmissions were and are yet unfolding within their borders. In comparison to the developed nations named above, testing in Africa and Haiti still appears to be insufficient for optimal containment.

It was also evident in Africa and Haiti that rapid increases in confirmed cases and hospitalizations were overpowering the weak public health and clinical care services. These already fragile public health and clinical care systems, lacking vital equipment to test and deliver prompt results and staff to address positive results, were bracing for greater numbers of sick people over the course of several months.

Testing people for COVID-19 has been shown to be crucial in helping to both diagnose individuals, and to understand how broadly the virus proliferated. Identifying who was infected and where they lived would have allowed health professionals and services to plan and deal with the demand for intensive care units. Testing could also help inform decisions on whether to narrow or soften prevention and mitigation measures.

Testing in any disease environment, and more especially in the case of COVID-19, is crucial in the larger public health picture as a mitigation effort, assisting researchers in the characterization of the pervasiveness, spread, and contagiousness of a disease. If testing reveals that a significant number of the population has already been infected, lockdown and other preventive and mitigative measures might not have to be so rigorous. Testing may also be an indicator of the effectiveness of self-quarantine, which could also inform whether or not the population would be ready to return to employment.

Throughout the pandemic as the demand for more testing was put forth by scientists, governments, and public health officials, there was a further complexity as they had to caution about the shortfalls of testing supplies, rising demand, and lengthy delays for results, and how these prevented possible contact-tracing attempts in places with serious surges.

Testing for the virus had (and has) an additional benefit: it provided some peace of mind to people if they tested negative, that they were not carrying the disease and therefore did not have to worry about possibly spreading it among family, friends, and community. Some people did not feel compelled to get tested and even claimed it was ethically inappropriate to be tested if they were asymptomatic and not at high risk. However, because the disease was challenging to control and because many asymptomatic people unknowingly spread it, more testing would have helped discover hidden cases and even now could still be effective in determining hotspots of contagion.

Knowing one's infection status helped with another key area

impacted by the virus: those with immunity could safely return to and continue working in key surroundings such as health care, public safety, and the service industries. They could also work in "non-essential" locations with less demand for critical personal protection equipment, which could be more serviceable for front-line health care providers.

Mass testing was deemed important to trace and contain the pandemic, as unlike other developed nations, many African countries and Haiti still did not have accurate data on infection rates. Such large-scale testing also served to support health services in better identifying and isolating the infected and co-ordinating their care, which helps to decelerate transmission and can help prevent unexpected spikes across communities and countries, thereby diminishing overall numbers of cases.

Effective testing and isolation approaches contribute to easing the burden on health services, which, in some countries, experienced a deluge of critical patients whose needs for care placed major demands for surge medical practices, staffing, respirators, ventilators, and other lifesaving equipment.

From a clinical care standpoint, testing for seroconversion, (which is the technical term for going from non-infected to infected to immune) can also detect COVID-19 specific antibodies in the plasma of those who were infected. This plasma could be used for infusions to treat the infected and avoid acute complications. This approach, using such plasma of those who have seroconverted, known as convalescent plasma, is not new; it was a therapeutic approach used during the 1918 flu pandemic.[163-165] The use of convalescent plasma in Africa and Haiti may be a way to unlock the COVID-19 puzzle, help people with compromised immune systems, essential workers, and older people to be safer and to defeat it.

According to the World Health Organization (WHO), two types of tests were used to identify the infection.[166] One, the PCR test (polymerase chain reaction test), is a molecular approach that can detect extremely minute amounts of viral nucleic acids with high accuracy from any biological sample.

The diagnosis of infectious diseases has been revolutionized by PCR. To reduce the inherent disadvantage of cost and improve the diagnostic efficiency of the test, multiplex PCR, a variant of the analysis in which one target sequence is strengthened using a pair of primers, has been improved.

A PCR test for the virus can be performed with a throat swab and establishes if one has the virus right then. PCR testing is the recommended test for diagnosing acute infection. Importantly, with PCR and DNA sequencing, the sources of most any virus can be traced, and scientists can establish how the virus was passed from one person to the next or from animals to people.

The second test is the antibody test. It received increased consideration as it can establish if people have been infected with the disease and their bodies successfully fought it off. Antibody tests do not detect the SARS-CoV2 virus that causes COVID-19 but rather, detects antibodies to the virus from a past infection.

Antibody tests are not suggested for diagnosing acute infection – meaning that they cannot detect if someone has the virus in the moment, but only that they had been exposed to it at some point in the past. Some antibody tests are less specific and will detect antibodies to other types of coronaviruses that cause the common cold and not COVID-19. It is inconclusive at this writing if having COVID-19 antibodies actually provides lasting immunity from reinfection.

There have been studies which suggest that people testing positive for antibodies might have a lower risk for future infections and some may even have some lifelong antibody protection. [167] One study asserts it found those who've had mild cases of the virus actually are more likely to acquire lifelong immunity as some antibody cells (called long-lived plasma cells) migrate to the bone marrow where they continue to produce and release into the bloodstream, low levels of antibodies.[168] Research led by the National Cancer Institute states that those presenting with prior SARS-CoV-2 infection "appear to have some degree of protection against being reinfected with the virus."[169] In light of opposing study findings there is no certainty as to whether or not SARS-CoV-2 antibodies confer long-term or short-term immunity.

Regarding the efficacy of the PCR and antibody tests, both may have false-positive results if one has had recent exposure.

In the case of the antibody test, a positive result – meaning antibodies are present - may not be generated for one to three weeks after exposure. The antibody test is, however, a better test to establish the infection rate within a community, and if conducted in sufficient numbers of the population, can be used as an infection rate indicator for entire countries.[170] Although considered a good indication of community infection rate, not everyone exposed to any virus, including the SARS-Cov-2, will produce detectable amounts of antibodies.[171-172] Of importance to viral spread is that both asymptomatic and those who do not produce detectable antibodies in the presence of disease, can still transmit the virus to others.

Findings from point-of-care tests may be accessed at the testing location in less than an hour. Other viral tests must be forwarded to a laboratory for analysis, a process that can take several days.

The bottom line is that as COVID-19 ravaged nations around the globe, increased testing was necessary before social distancing and mask wearing mandates could be eased or lifted entirely. However, as Africa and Haiti have a combined population of over 1.352 billion, testing everyone would not be realistic in a short period. A random sampling of a representative population country-wide, however, could have provided legitimate data on how widespread the infection was during the height of the pandemic and can be used even now for the same purpose.

It is recognized that youth and those under 60 may have exposure to the virus but be asymptomatic. What governments and health specialists do not know even now is how many within this sub-population are carrying the disease. That information could provide them a more accurate picture of individual exposure. Such data is essential in reestablishing normal activity, work, shopping, and recreation. The lack of this information as countries re-open their communities and borders lends to the false belief that caution has been well applied and successful, when in fact, the truth may be otherwise. Testing has proven to be an essential part of the approach to preventing COVID-19 from taking hold again by ensuring that it is not propagated across communities and countries.

While much of the focus of COVID-19 testing has been on diagnostic testing, antibody, or serology tests, there is a segment of the population that resists being tested because of rumors and misleading information that the swabs used to test for the virus are infected. Reluctance to be tested is not unique to most people living in "hotspots", but also to returned travelers who have so far not been affected by the virus and have been living relatively "normal" lives elsewhere.

Resistance and outright refusal to be tested was and remains an issue along with also resisting vaccination. When a sizable population refuses medical testing (if they have symptoms) or screening (if no symptoms) of any type it is usually because they want to avoid facing the diagnosis of a positive result and all that implies. Alternatively, they want to avert the perceived burden of the test procedure itself. There were (and still are) others who refuse testing because of long standing mistrust of the medical and scientific communities; while others resist for personal reasons and even fear that being tested could somehow hurt them or their children.

Many people also felt unprepared and cautious about door-knocking testing campaigns. It did not help that arguments about the origin and continuing spread of COVID-19 led to social stigma, discrimination, and marginalization, blame and ostracism. There were those who believed health systems were being used to convey the message that testing was mandatory. People balked at even the hint of mandatory testing as an infringement upon their rights and bodily integrity, insisting only they could decide what happens to their bodies without outside coercion – especially from government sponsored authorities.

Within Haiti and Africa, it has been revealed that the refusal to be tested is a direct consequence of the fact that their populations are facing considerable problems as there is no wide-ranging and/or long-term COVID-19 relief assistance extended to the population and primarily, to a large work force struggling with unemployment and beaten economies.

A workforce consisting almost entirely of independent entrepreneurs is a workforce without sick leave that would find itself under a considerable burden having to quarantine while waiting for test results which take several days. If people cannot attend work, their businesses close, or they may lose their jobs and important income altogether. Some held the hope that Haitian and African governments would provide some relief assistance and public servants would receive some special protection and equipment against exposure to the virus, but those hopes were dashed as these governments struggled to fund, allocate, and provide even the most basic of services in light of the pandemic.

Potential government programs intended to keep millions afloat since the start of the pandemic, coupled with continual financial hardship, have never been comprehensively enacted or extended to everyone. Against this backdrop of resistance and uncertainty there was also a profound belief that hospitals and health care facilities were high-risk hotspots for COVID-19 and should be avoided. These factors coalesced becoming justifications against testing so as to avoid not working and thereby losing income while awaiting test results.

Some evidence has been presented that the facilities of a few African countries were and are safe, accessible, approachable to all members of the public. There have been a few reports of a substantial attempts having been made to make it faster and easier to test, but people refused and are still rebuffing health facilities, especially test labs, because they believe they will become infected once there. This fear has its basis in the perception that once there is a pandemic, all healthcare institutions become central reservoirs of the virus because sick people always go to those facilities. This belief and accompanying behaviors were common prior to the COVID-19 pandemic but became more pronounced especially in the beginning and at the apex of the pandemic. People need to understand that hospital and clinic facilities were and are still functioning primarily as care institutions for patients who have other medical complications and conditions, not just infectious diseases. Public health officials and medical practitioners should do all they can to dispel the opinion that hospitals are reservoirs of mass infection.

Reluctance to be tested was also revealed to be prevalent among a larger number of persons recognized as close contacts of confirmed cases. This group refused to present for testing, despite it being offered free of charge if they came forward. This reticence was based in fear of having been exposed to the virus and feelings of being distrusted, embarrassed, and stigmatized in a critical period when they needed a hand to support them. Also, they were worried about missing rent, losing their housing, jobs, a paycheck, and their relationships if they took time off to quarantine. Further, a persistent distrust of the government and public health services caused people who contracted COVID-19 to deny sharing information about close contacts before they tested positive, while others have rejected out of perceived disgrace.

It has not helped that close contacts of confirmed cases have not been reliable as they claimed to have not been in contact with anyone, although evidence showed they were living in the same house with several infected people.

Some countries introduced punishments, the extension of hotel quarantine, and the prospective for fines for those unwilling to take part in the testing processes. In retaliation, people expressed their resentment by saying that forced testing was not the best course of action as it would produce an antagonistic and distrustful relationship with the government and public health services since COVID-19 is not the only infectious disease emergency people will experience. If governments would remove obstacles to taking part in public health activities, in the immediate and long term, and develop reliable public health services, this could empower people to follow health regulations and would establish an enduring public good.

Another factor that has affected successful testing is the lack of reliable transport or money for transportation to get to a testing facility. This reality demands that governments and public health services establish testing sites and campaigns around hotspots and in rural areas – this could ease peoples' movement.

The hosting of pop-up sites at varying locations should be established. Public health messaging should encourage people to get tested with a coherent message to dispel any fear or misinformation about the virus and the testing methods and protocols. It is crucial to emphasize the fact that infected people are sent to isolation facilities where they are given proper treatment so as not to infect others. Messaging that highlights that effective measures have been enacted across communities and countries to prevent continued transmission of the virus should be created and shared across and throughout Haiti and the nations of Africa.

It has been brought to light that governments and public health providers have not done enough to reach linguistically diverse communities and populations, which could be a substantial problem. Through no fault of their own, there are people who live in remote and rural areas along with others who do not speak or understand (very well) the national language. They, therefore, may not be receiving COVID-19 health advice about symptoms, isolation, or testing needs.

Government and public health providers, unequivocally, need to understand why most people reject testing and improve public health approaches to testing that support and encourage people to make decisions that are in the public and the country's best interests.

Substantial challenges are facing many African countries, the USVI, and Haiti as they attempt to increase COVID-19 testing to the recommended levels; central among these is the significant scarcity of available testing sites and equipments.

In nations such as Mauritius, Australia, Taiwan, and South Korea, where the pandemic appears to have slowed its progression and life is being set to some level of past normalcy, the accomplishment of these countries shows the key to pandemic control lies in early aggressive strategizing of approaches. These included strict testing regimens, a staunch and operable plan for isolation and quarantine of the infected, cooperation of the population based in concern for others (beneficence), enforcement of preventive and mitigation measures that include regulated shopping for necessities, defined transportation, masks, and quarantine in designated supervised spaces to limit exposure to strangers, family, and friends.

As with managing any scarce resource, first, Africa and Haiti's governments and public health authorities should prioritize where to roll out testing to have the most effect, and second, they must commit to accomplishing this delivery properly and promptly. Public service announcements and campaigns which use the language of the local people, and which speak to their sensibilities - protection of themselves, their children, keeping their jobs – should be developed and disseminated.

Essential workers who may yet be reluctant to be tested and vaccinated, should also be targeted with messaging that speaks to their daily concerns: being able to continue working in a healthy way; not spreading disease to their families, and being able to continue providing for their families.

COVID-19 Conspiracy Theories Spread on Social Media Put 'Everyone' at Risk

COVID-19 has grown into the largest and most problematic public health challenge of a generation fraught with an overabundance of misinformation. One essential factor that actually helped spur the deluge of misinformation, conspiracy theories, myths, and outright falsehoods was one of the very measures enacted to help mitigate spread of the virus: mandatory lockdowns.

With people sequestered indoors for months, shifting to the internet as a source of news became a norm, placing social media front and center as a resource. Within this virtual environment a significant overflow of misinformation and conspiracy theories were circulated placing "everyone" at risk as these increased people's mistrust and doubt in the systems established to help them. Even those who did not, and do not even now believe the stories and conspiracies, cannot help but be influenced to some degree by what they read and see on the internet. In this way, social media has become the purveyor of insidious untruths having far-reaching consequences.

Unfortunately, there were and are no readily available panaceas to stem the tides of the mushrooming outbreak of coronavirus misinformation, conspiracy theories, hoaxes, anti-mask myths, anti-social distancing, anti-testing, and gross inaccuracies surrounding the efficacy of vaccinations, or fake treatments. Public doubts around the scientific process, combined with growing frustrations with lockdown restrictions and struggling economies, formed a suitable storm in which gross inaccuracies were, and are yet, flourishing.

In previous public health emergency responses such as Ebola, Dengue Fever, and HIV/AIDS, social media was used to encourage people to take precautionary measures and informed health professionals of anyone showing symptoms. Important local information was distributed freely on social media to help people confront disease and protect themselves and their loved ones. Many of these same efforts are taking place now but are being eclipsed on a larger scale by messaging with the distinctive purpose of swaying people from listening to public authorities and instead, encouraging them to follow their own dictates of conscience – be they right or wrong, helpful, or destructive.

It has been purported in the past that African nations and Haiti were among the "lost countries" of the information technology (IT) age because they were the least computerized and the most lacking in infrastructure to support IT advances. But today, they are fastly reaching levels of usage and virtual presence similar to that of more developed nations, especially where the use of social media is concerned. And despite the diverging aging populations and cultures, there has been a substantial gain in social networking sites usage over the preceding decades among all age groups.

Ample evidence has revealed that across nations, young people (18 to 36 years) alongside the more highly educated, are more likely to use online social networking sites such as Facebook, Google, LinkedIn, WhatsApp, Microsoft, Tic Tök, Yahoo Reddit, Twitter, and YouTube. Similarly, it has been shown that social media platforms are used by individuals of different literacy abilities, and this helped people not only to gain access to information about COVID-19 prevention approaches but also facilitated the transmission of communication to vulnerable populations living in remote localities.

Granted, online social platforms have been demonstrated to be of major value as appealing tools for health communication and information dissemination, but they have also been a primary source for exposing large swaths of populations to falsehoods and conspiracy theories. This readiness and willingness to seek information online has been spurred by a need to get clarity when the messages of governments and public health officials, at times, appeared contradictory, and even inaccurate.

The proliferation of mass misinformation about COVID-19 via the virtual world became known as "*infodemic*", a term that was quickly added to the website, dictionary.com.

According to the site, "An *infodemic* is defined as an overload of information, often false or unverified, about a problem, especially a major crisis. Quickly spreading in the news, online, and through social media, this information fuels fear and speculation, making the problem worse, not better."[173]

Concurrence with this definition was given by the World Health Organization describing *infodemics* as "an excessive amount of information about a problem which makes it difficult to identify a solution. They can spread misinformation, disinformation, and rumor's during a health emergency. *Infodemics* can hamper an effective public health response and create confusion and distrust among people."[174]

While most of the world's populations have been engaged to support their country's safety, a sizable group of people still believe COVID-19 is a political and worldwide hoax to manipulate people. Such disinformation/misinformation hides healthy behaviors and encourages fallacious practices that raise the spread of the virus and lead to poor physical and mental health consequences among people. Falsehoods and conspiracy theories also lead to rising deterioration of the information context, a distrust of knowledge, scientists, and the main conception of accuracy.

Although some misinformation and conspiracy theories can (at times) be harmless, they have struck a nerve and helped the radicalization of fringe groups. This rather sizable group of people has joined one of the self-reinforcing cohorts of the collectively unhinged, which have become abnormally popular in the generation of social media. Most of these radicalized nonbelievers produce an absolute public health risk as they have been less willing to follow social distancing measures, wearing a face mask or proper cloth face, and have been less prone to be tested, and resist vaccination. Public health specialists around the world were afraid that the surge of unpleasant information on social media platforms was undermining efforts to slow the virus, and they have substantiated reasons to believe this.

Studies led by scientists at McGill University in Montreal have established that "people who have their news from social media platforms like Facebook, Google, LinkedIn, Microsoft, WhatsApp, Tip Tök, Yahoo Reddit, Twitter, and YouTube are more likely to have misperceptions about COVID-19." In addition, the study found that the vast majority of misinformation came from a singular national source: the United States of America, where the attitude of personal rights was touted to take precedence over coalescing as a united people to save the lives of hundreds of thousands of their own people and others around the globe.[175-176]

Another instance of risks imputable to inappropriate health

communication through social media platforms can found in Nigeria, where health care providers discovered many cases of overdose of chloroquine (a medication used to treat malaria) following news on the alleged efficacy of the medicine for treating COVID-19 transmission through the social media.[177]

The prevalence of disinformation associated with the diagnosis and therapy of COVID-19 has perplexed both the general population and healthcare providers, who are struggling with a relatively under-studied virus. These falsities and conspiracy theories enhanced local suspicions and caused bitterness toward and mistrust of foreign health workers and NGOs.

These angels of mercy found themselves the victims of torrid verbal attacks and their access to testing sites and tracing blocked. The hoaxes and disinformation also produced a social stigma around COVID-19, which led to decreased conformity with stay-at-home, masking, and social distancing orders as people found themselves ridiculed, and in the cases of store, restaurant, and airplane employees, physically attacked for compliance and enforcement of mitigation guidelines and employer regulations.

Many countries have recounted incidents where hundreds of people were infected by a single individual who visited their mosque or church despite their doctor's recommendation to stay isolated at the house.[178] Such inconveniences subsidize the suboptimal management of the COVID-19 outbreak across various populations. This further diminishes the validity of new scientific conclusions for proposed cures or vaccines for this disease.

While developed countries may have powers, experiences, and approaches to oppose health-related misinformation and conspiracy theories, this is much more challenging in many African countries, the USVI, and Haiti as governments and local public health experts are often negatively perceived among the populous and appear to be unreliable sources of information about COVID-19. In fact, some misinformation and conspiracy theories blame governments and public health specialists for having set COVID-19 in motion in order to gain access to aid money or to secure votes in elections. Other conspiracy theories asserted that COVID-19 was somehow sent to poorer countries on purpose by Westerners who were exploring approaches to infect people for the purpose of extermination.

The mainstreaming of misreported information and conspiracy theories about the start and transmission of the virus seriously complicated the ability to handle the pandemic by further eroding the public's tendency to adhere to public health guidance. However, being aware of the various conspiracy theories and myths can help inform those in authority about the mindsets of people and societies where such misinformation originates and proliferates. Knowledge about these groups can help inform how to design better messaging that effectively combats the impacts of inaccurate information.

It is imperative that we also view this pandemic and the proliferation of misinformation in a historical context. In the instance of every plague and deadly disease, there have been misinformation and conspiracy theories to explain their source and how to, hypothetically, prevent their transmission. Often, those falsehoods and theories play on worries prevailing within the cultural surroundings at the time. For example, HIV/AIDS denialists, people who believed that HIV did not cause AIDS, were reacting not just to AIDS, but to the context of AIDS in these countries especially in the African continent of the 1980s, where the epidemic appeared to wipe out the most exposed and neglected in society with little consideration or care from mainstream authority and leaders. This led to people having even less trust in the systems which they felt had suppressed them and lied to them, and which were now needed to save their lives.

Africa and Haiti are experiencing some parallel dynamics playing out in the present. The range of misinformation and falsehoods further reveals particular strands of widespread beliefs about power in these areas today.

In a period of staggering socioeconomic disparity where coronavirus is exposing the life-or-death stakes of that disparity, the rise of misinformation and conspiracy theories within the African continent, the USVI, and Haiti suggesting the disease is a scheme by elites to gain profit and authority, should not be surprising. Our field assessment results, paired with unpublished surveys, established that a sizable population within these areas perceived at least some credibility in the falsities that the COVID-19 pandemic was plotted by prominent elites.

Our assessment surveys discovered that most people appear

not to have substantial faith in their public broadcast stations' competence to provide facts about the disease. Instead, they relied on friends, families, and social media platforms. The survey further revealed that most people commonly have considerably more confidence in social media platforms than their local television news and newspapers.

As the pandemic raged on throughout 2020, confidence in science and health was sorely tested as fringe groups - politically and socially motivated – forged ahead pushing misinformation with the result of diminishing the numbers of those complying with preventive behaviors. Many found themselves not complying because of uncertainty and confusion as to the veracity of any available information.

The reality is that misinformation and conspiracy theories about disease outbreaks will always take place. It is, however, the responsibility of government leadership and health authorities tasked with telling the truth and sharing facts, to avoid giving a platform to dubious claims that have no grounding in reality, and to set about rigorously disproving those claims through conscientious and factual clarification.

It is unambiguous that people living in confinement, or under threat of a contagious disease outbreak suffer psychosocial stress and damaging health effects which may spur their interest in learning more about the disease or virus. However, such circumstances need assurance supplemented by a flow of accurate and verifiable information.

This necessity has been recognized by the WHO, which has collaborated with the leadership of many of the social media platforms and major tech companies to remove rumors and disinformation, alongside promoting important new revisions from healthcare institutions.[179] While social media platforms are a double-edged sword, they can be employed to disseminate efficient science and health communication. It would also be helpful if those crafting scientific and health-based information messages would be aware of how dispersed information is perceived.

To successfully improve the dissemination of facts and truthful information and counter the deluge of gross misinformation, several strategies must be employed.

First, the virtual world via the internet and the use of online video combines many benefits for science and health communication. It functions on a visual and an auditory level. This implies that a variety of spoken local languages, including a diverse set of captions, could be used. People who have difficulty reading or are sight compromised will be able to use and understand information delivered via audio. Yet, caution must be applied as it is well known that the primary online video-sharing platform, YouTube, is known for being used to propagate misinformation and conspiracy theories.[180] Therefore, governments and public health specialists should be encouraged to consider the extraordinary potential of the online video format for science and health communication purposes, particularly during local public health crises and also to counter rumors, misconceptions, and all types of misinformation.

Second, mass media such as (radio, newspaper, magazines, television, radio), community agencies, assistance groups, and civil society could play important functions in publicizing truthful information. To carry this out, it is vital to develop strategic collaborations at local and country levels, linking offline and online resources in a coordinated approach so that confirmed information is transmitted across media platforms.

Third, all hoaxes and rumors must be deleted from all online media platforms, and these sources must agree to approve and only publish and allow the publication of scientifically viable and verified information to raise awareness among the population at large. Innovative technologies such as natural language controlling, or text-mining methods may be beneficial in identifying online media content that has no scientific or health basis. The latest data-mining algorithms have proven effective at uncovering the particular features of all forms of bogus news and deleting them from their associated platforms.[181] Twitter, Reddit, and Amazon have already applied these approaches to delete fake accounts or product evaluations. Application of these same principles to end all rumors and hoaxes about the COVID-19 outbreak is therefore clearly achievable.

Fourth, there should be regulations and legal ramifications for online platforms that allow production and dissemination of such disinformation, and also for the people who post the misinformation. Local and national supervisory agencies and law enforcement agencies should be informed of these issues to address them. There is evidence that governments of some countries have apprehended people engaged in the distribution of such disinformation.[182]

However, before implementing any of these laws, authorities in Africa, the USVI and Haiti's should carry out a proper review and make sure of the lawful rights of the suspects.

Fifth, common platforms should be launched to offer preventative information in both online and offline media to a general substantial extent. Effective approaches for mass media campaigns from the last few epidemics such as Ebola and HIV/AIDS should be identified and applied. These mass media promotions should be culturally customized and translated into many languages based in each country's diversity context to increase outreach.

Sixth, telemedicine should offer evidence-based care and informational services that are accessible to individuals with restricted access to care, such as people living in remote and rural areas, the aged, and those who are just stranded in their homes because of a lockdown order. This will both decrease the threat of hospital-acquired illnesses, and also lessen the use of resources such as ventilators and personal protective equipment (PPE) for frontline health providers.

Lastly, clarity, excellent information management, and leadership across communities and organizations should be encouraged to end false information about COVID-19. This is vital for the greater good for people suffering from the health and psychosocial burdens of this outbreak.

One last note regarding the issue of information dissemination via virtual platforms: There exists a secondary infodemic created by the stories, myths, preconceptions, and superstitions that proliferate within various cultures and are spread person-to person, generation to generation. This type of infodemic is more difficult to fight and to dampen because it has its roots in long-standing strong cultural beliefs that are shared and published without any editorial oversight, and they do not fall under any realm of control or authority to stem them.

One way to stem the tide of such storytelling as it relates to disease information is to employ persons from the tribes, villages, and localities, train them in the proper health messaging and have them meet with village and local leaders. If the person is known or has family ties in the area, they are less likely to be shunned and what they say will have more sway. If tribal, village and religious leaders can be brought on board to share correct and informative messaging, they will be the strongest allies to stopping the spread of "stories" and misinformation.

Lack of Effective Safety Net Pushed People to Disregard Strict Preventive measures.

In the face of the COVID-19 pandemic, the African continent, the USVI, and Haiti along with many nations around the world established strict lockdown measures that shut down all formal and informal businesses, commercial properties, tourism, hospitality services, and mass gatherings without enough mitigation approaches to relieve the impacts this would have on the afflicted populations and households. These preventive measures, although necessary, proved to be the source of unbearable economic trauma, heightened stress, and dysfunction within families and relationships. In many African countries no safety net was considered or provided; while in Haiti, it was not financially possible to provide a safety net.

In the United States people responded with panic, storming through store aisles buying up massive amounts of paper goods (toilet paper, paper towels, wipes, etc.), dry goods food items, and cleaning supplies. This was not the case in African countries where the opportunity to make mass purchases of this type were limited to on-hand supplies. The same was true for Haiti and even the USVI where much of what is needed on these islands is brought in by boat and plane, thereby limiting on-hand stores of goods. Thus, the major fear that enveloped the populations of these areas was the failure of mainly impoverished people to stock up on food and other essentials for survival over the course of the lockdown period. This dearth of ample food and other supplies was notoriously noted in a video from Lagos, Nigeria showing people shouting about the famine that cannot be remediated because of the lockdown.[183]

This reaction in Nigeria was not uncommon in other countries. A United Nations study found that more than 150 million children became impoverished due to COVID-19 restrictions on movement, business closures, lost wages and jobs, and overall shrinking economies.

The countries of Cambodia, Uganda, India, Kenya, El Salvador, the Philippines, and many others reported dire consequences upon the poor, the elderly, and children due to the restrictions to thwart the tide of the pandemic. Added to this picture of famine and poverty was increased violence levied by police and other authoritarian figures charged to enforce the lockdowns and waged against these same poor who, out of desperation, were compelled to break the rules of quarantine and lockdowns to find ways to earn what meager wages they could to feed themselves and their families, to provide care and daily necessities.[184-190]

For the indigent who are without the comfort of bank savings or credit cards, public health efforts that slashed their means of regular revenue seemed to provide an antidote that was as awful as the virus itself. Given these damaging outcomes, it became morally questionable to restrict people from functioning without affording them a way to care for their elementary demands.

Poor people and low-income laborers have felt the effect of

the pandemic the toughest because of systemic economic and health inequalities. Even before the COVID-19 shutdowns caused massive job losses, household poverty had exploded, people's financial delinquencies were rising, and many did not have money to provide for potential emergency expenses.

The one segment of the poor who were spared food shortages were farmers who produced most of their own food. Survival farming, a burden in normal periods due to its minimal production, represents an autonomy and self-dependence that helped small farmers escape the trading limitations brought about because of COVID-19.

Similarly, paid urban laborers, most of whom serve governments or state-owned industries, were experiencing serious financial crunches as the delivery of food supplies became strained and price inflation in markets or stores rose steeply.

Informal traders and entrepreneurs without prior support, found themselves spending most of their days breaking lockdown mandates to conduct business as best they could with the expectation of generating revenue to support their families. Day-to-pay laborers – people who work and are paid for their day's labor and may or may not have work the next day – were exceptionally hard hit by the mandatory lockdowns in less developed nations, with Africa and Haiti taking enormous economic hits within this group.[191, 192] Self-operating and family-owned small businesses in sectors such as wholesale, embroidery, handicraft manufacturing, and taxicab/motorcycle passenger services, make up more than two-thirds of urban work in these countries according to our field assessment paired with unpublished surveys.[193] In Africa and Haiti millions of people and their relatives depend on salaries from these businesses and were doubtful of being able to survive a lockdown for more than a week. In Haiti there were additional problems involving the informal trade industry, micro-entrepreneurs, and efforts to thwart the rising tide of COVID-19 cases.

Many of Haiti's citizens have yet to recover from the impacts of the 2010 earthquake and thus have not had stable housing and reliable access to clean water and sanitary conditions, with the vast majority being impoverished, residing in close-quartered camp-like settlements, and eeking out a living via informal trade mechanisms. This scenario is a ripe environment for the rapid transmission of diseases, viruses, and any other contagious anomaly.

Added to this backdrop was that school-age children were unable to continue their education because there was insufficient IT infrastructure to take classes on-line. This meant there was a greater likelihood of the young acquiring the virus, possibly being asymptomatic, and passing it on to adults and the elderly also residing in those encampments, thereby, boosting the propensity for disease proliferation and further complicating efforts to control viral spread.

That Haiti's government had no initial pandemic response plan in place and did not have the financial resources to provide its citizens with temporary income support, has helped to fuel a more grim and uncertain future in the face of the pandemic for the tiny island nation.

Placing salt in the already seething wounds of its poor, the government itself dealt a hard blow to the informal traders and micro-entrepreneurs when it chose to keep the marketplaces where they conduct business under mandatory closure, but reopened foreign-owned, operated, and supported sweatshop businesses and textile factories as early as April 2020. People felt the government had once again acted in a manner that demonstrated a blatant disregard for its citizens favoring the financial gains to the government over saving the lives and livelihoods of its own people, adding to the mounting distrust between the two.[194, 195]

Food insecurity also played a major role in compliance to public health mandates for COVID-19. Millions of Haitians are food insecure, lack access to clean water, lack electricity, and starvation and malnutrition are constant realities. In this new pandemic world hunger is more severe as unemployment and loss of wages and work opportunities made it increasingly difficult to provide food for families.[196, 197]

Housing also fell under the wicked spell of COVID-19 impacts. The prerogative of owning a house is emphasized by governments everywhere, and during COVID regulations were put in place which enabled mortgage payments to be suspended for qualified homeowners; but no comparable policy measures were promulgated to postpone rent disbursements, leaving renters without a viable safety net.

In the USVI, which is a territory of the United States, the moratorium on evictions was granted in 2020 and extended in May 2021, but that did not stop some landlords from still evicting tenants. Of greater importance is that the moratorium did not provide for or address what will happen when it is lifted, and people still do not have jobs and sufficient savings or income to pay any back-owed rent. This lack will make them vulnerable to being evicted, so the moratorium is just stalling the inevitable. Mass evictions mean increased numbers of homeless, which means another and different type of drain on the social fabric of the islands where the cost of living is growing higher each year as wealthy expats flock to the islands making it their home causing prices to go up and the availability of land on which to build to diminish.

While these economic strategies might have been helpful for a time, they were just stopgap measures for some people and unlikely to have any permanent effect on the key social factors of health. Similar to the curative health system approaches, they are reactive, not proactive and curative to some degree, but definitely not preventive. This implies that many of the measures designed to ameliorate some of the stressors caused by COVID-19 may not have been adequately carried out since there were no suitably legislated social safety net policies in place to assure they were effective and enforced.

The bottom line here is that for the populations of Africa

and Haiti, compliance to public health mandates was in fact for many, the kiss of death. Without adequate housing, access to fresh running water and sanitation, coupled with a mandate to remain indoors and not work, many already struggling and malnourished families would lose loved ones not to COVID-19 directly, but indirectly due to its exacerbation of pre-existing life and health threatening conditions.

Another important piece in this discussion is the direct role of governments in protecting and watching out for the best interests of their citizenry.

Many of these countries, particularly in the African continent, have a longstanding record of stringent measures being created and enforced upon informal businesses during an emergency such as COVID-19.[198] Police and military enforcement of mandates only served to further disenfranchise and even criminalize people on the brink of annihilation and desperate to live out the same benefits and privileges as the elite and well-to-do within their societies, but without the means to do so unless they exercised non-compliance to the COVID-19 restrictions, thereby, breaking the law.

The helplessness and disintegration of these groups illustrates the disparity and inequities between those of wealth and means and the poor. It also shows us how the focus of a government can make or break its own people through policy and legislation. Unlike developed countries such as the United States of America, where the emphasis is on comprehensive economic stimulus packages for expansive remediation and response to the impacts of the pandemic, in lesser developed nations the urgent emphasis has been on immediate disaster assistance and maintaining control at any and all costs.

Poorer nations that did attempt economy-centered strategies, sadly, were lacking in facts and determination, as the proportions of the financial packages were largely insignificant and therefore, incapable of meeting the needs of the populous.[199] Countries such as Ethiopia put together a proposed relief package that was just 0.15 percent of GDP, while Rwanda's strong package amounted to 1.5 percent of GDP. By comparison, the amounts of the U.S. stimulus package corresponded to 10 percent of GDP. In oil-supplying countries such as Nigeria, Angola, and Gabon, huge budget shortfalls affected by the unparalleled oil cost collapse hampered governments' ability to propose an effective assistance package.[200, 201]

The facts presented here are an ardent statement of demand and need that Haiti and the nations of Africa, and the USVI promptly put together or reinforce social safety net packages that focus on informal businesses and other exposed economic groups such as day-pay workers. Wherever practical, they must promote honest micro-credit mechanisms and tax exemptions to enhance the ability of micro-entrepreneurs and informal business workers to achieve financial parity. While many of these informal sectors are not in government registries and the status of their activities is unproven, restricting their ability to survive does not benefit the national economy and pushes people further into poverty creating a heavier burden for the nation.

Effective programs that incorporate financial assistance or immediate supply for crucial commodities such as food, fuel, and electricity, alongside a decrease in payments for essential services related to phone, internet, banking, and rent should be enforced. Enforcing moratoria on the real estate or rental income taxes could likewise have advantageous outcomes for many of these small-scale businesses that use leased areas. Another improvement that would be of help to people in severe economic straits or confronting health emergencies would be the development and implementation of universal free health insurance.

The COVID-19 disaster presents an unparalleled opportunity for governments to engage systematic attempts to digitize, register, and coordinate informal sectors, and make available vital services to assist them in being successful. For instance, supporting the launching of standard or mobile-based bank accounts, which could decrease the operational challenge of organizing rescue fund transfers at the last mile.[202] Parallel initiatives that reinforce the survival ability of micro-businesses could enhance their readiness to deal with forthcoming disasters.

Although as of this writing many nations are reopening businesses and lifting restrictions on public activities and even mask wearing, the cruel reality is that there were pandemics and epidemics before COVID-19, and there will be more after, and the protocols set in place now will be needed when the next one occurs. Therefore, governments must discuss and plan for relief for their citizens for without adequate relief for informal businesses and the urban underprivileged, social distancing restrictions and other preventive measures designed to prevent a pandemic from taking hold, will completely fall apart.

For public health prevention efforts to be effective, African countries, the USVI, and Haitian governments and public health specialists must respond promptly to reformulate emergency social safety net incentives that provide support to those harshly touched by the economic lockdown, and the planning and approach must be from the perspective of not 'if a pandemic or disaster occurs,' but 'when another pandemic or disaster occurs.'

CHAPTER FOUR

Real Life Impact of Rumors and Misinformation on COVID-19

Note: We have already discussed the types of rumors, misinformation, myths, and conspiracy theories that prevailed throughout the COVID-19 pandemic, and in many places still prevail. In this chapter, using the words and experiences of actual persons encountered during our assessments, we aim to demonstrate just how insidious and damaging this malicious and protracted rumor mill can affect life and death decisions.

The following scenes are relayed in the exact words of the persons interviewed.

Except for persons who voluntarily consented to be identified, names of individuals have been changed for considerations of privacy.

Selected COVID-19 Rumors and Misinformation

James Funsah Abayomi, 39, Driver; Douala, Cameroon

If I had not come to the hospital, I would most likely have died. I work as a driver in Douala Cameroon. I had a fever for nearly four weeks before going to the hospital. My wife and one of my two children also had a fever, but they healed more rapidly than me. I took traditional medicines made from oak leaves, lilacs, and aloe vera prescribed by friends to take care of myself at home. At first, I did not believe I had COVID-19, because I had not been in close contact with people from abroad, so I did not think I could get infected.

When my health condition did not get better, a friend and my wife wanted to call the ambulance to take me to the nearest hospital, but I refused and getting upset with the craziest idea. These Days, as soon as people see an ambulance pass, they instantaneously believe the person inside has COVID-19, and on some occasion, they have even threatened people because of this.

As time passed, my health condition worsens significantly, including persistent bouts of bloody mucus when I was coughing, and I could not get up because I was losing my physical strength. Finally, my wife and best friend took me to the COVID-19 center in his private vehicle, to prevent causing fear in the community. If they had not taken me there even against my will then, I would probably have died. In my community, many people complain about experiencing a fever. They asserted they would instead die at home than going to the hospital because they were persuaded that hospital staff will inject them with a deadly vaccine. While I have been hospitalized, several relatives and friends have either texted or called me, to implore me not to accept injections. This rumor linked to vaccines is profoundly rooted in Cameroon. Lately, a friend I used to give a drive to his workplace was hospitalized with a cardiovascular disease condition, died days later, and people rumored it was because the hospital staff injected him with a vaccine, which was not true at all. I have been treated here for 14 days now and I am feeling better, and I hope to go home soon. So, based on my experience, I want to let people know that is important, that they feel fearless to go to the hospital or health care center and seek treatment once they have symptoms of fever or breathing problems. They should not be afraid of being stigmatized by relatives, friends, or community members around them.

Delyno Adams Fleming, 42, event planner; St Croix, U.S. Virgin Islands (USVI)

All my friends always believed that COVID-19 is a government hoax to seek international funding. After nearly several weeks of confinement, many people including some of my close relatives are suffering from mental fatigue. People I spoke with on the streets and others I do business with are in total agreement with me the imposed confinement and strict health recommendations such as stay home or to wear a face mask are illegal, and the authorities do not have the power to force them. No law or court endorses this view. Let us face it, this disease is a total scam, and the confirmed case numbers given daily are being counted more than once, leading to exaggerated numbers. For instance, a close relative intended to get tested for the virus, because he was planning to travel abroad, but never completed the test because of the long wait times, and later on, getting a letter showing he tested positive for COVID-19, so this story of COVID-19 virus is completely bogus. Could you have imagined how hard mentally, physically, and emotionally my friend was after reading the letter and how his close family reacted about all this fake news? Also, I read on social media that COVID-19, if it exists, which I doubt, is transmitted by contaminated testing swabs, and hospital staff are using patients with just a minor fever as bait for the COVID-19 vaccine experimentations. So, now I am more convinced that all this scam is not about helping or supporting the poor population here, but it is about attracting relief funding from abroad for their interests.

Koumba Mwune Ndinge, 38, health care professional; Libreville, Gabon

COVID-19 is fake, and it has not disturbed lives (my family and I) at all, and we are still doing tasks as normal. Although there is an assumption that people will follow, that they will take personal responsibility and avoid crowds, and keep a distance of public transport, many people, including myself, are yet living fearlessly and do not follow these rubbish health recommendations. Elsewhere, people are not so trusting of our government and public health's expertise in managing COVID-19, if it exists, and there is also a substantial skepticism about the case numbers they are telling the population.

Our country is not an exemplary model for mass diagnostic testing, therefore the so announced confirmed case and death numbers are just a way to put more fear into the population's mind as always. The real numbers are much lower, but they are making them higher to be eligible for COVID-19 Emergency Relief Fund given by the World Health Organization (WHO). Coronavirus (COVID-19) is not widely spread and has never been a threat for the population, except for the government and public health services which are spreading bogus information. COVID-19 is like the flu and social media messages and videos are showing us it is harmless. Therefore, people should continue to do what they want to do and enjoy their lives to the fullest.

Solange Azor Briscoe, 48, self-employed; Port-au-Prince, Haiti

One early afternoon, Solange Azor Briscoe, 48, was in her regular place close to a lottery stand near to the Champ of Mars, struggling to sell hot coffee, hot chocolate, bread, and some cold drinks. Although the government requested people to stay home and warned those who will not wear face masks or appropriate cloth face coverings with a fine of $300 which could represent half a year's salary for more than half the population who has been often spotted maskless. "If COVID-19 virus was in Haiti, it would have now claimed the lives of most people, who do not want to wear the face masks," she said. Not far away from her, Charles Petit Pierre, who moved several years ago from Cap-Haïtien to Pieton-Ville, was also trying to sell new and used books and some second-hand school supplies to students milling about, although the government closed all schools and universities. "Yes, I have overheard about this fake disease, it is in other countries, but here in Haiti, everybody has been lying about it. I do not trust the government, who only looks at making extra money on behalf of poor people" he said. And so, no wonder *that activists have scrawled graffiti-like "Where is the Corona relief money?" on walls, imitating the slogan from the last years' anti-bribery demonstrations: "Where is the Petrocaribe money?" People like Charles Petit Pierre "think rumors that say COVID-19 are a tall tale invented by the authorities suspected of corruption so they can attract financial aid from international donors." Solange Azor Briscoe and Charles Petit Pierre "claimed also not to be trusting of international humanitarian actors, whose repeated promises in the wake of the 2010 earthquake did not deliver the promised Haiti "build back better," instead are helping the authorities telling untruths about COVID-19 virus." They concluded by saying "before COVID-19 people always were sick and dying of "epidemic lafyèv" meaning fever epidemic, the authorities were doing nothing because money was not attached to it, now they are talking about it every day just to attract relief funding from abroad."*

Azagba Ekaghogho Housou, 30, health analyst; Porto Novo, Benin

There is this increase in the death rate. This is a very ordinary idea that the authorities use to take away liberty. They often take something that is a genuine risk, then hyper exaggerate it. They catastrophize it to provoke fear and panic, so that then whatever they do is justified. So, I believe it is not on the point where people should be in a state of fear. It is not as if COVID-19 is highly contagious. I recognize that there is an enormous amount of doubt about the deadliness of it, mainly since when they are computing the deadliness of it, what they are often doing is they are telling how many people are deceased, divided by how many diagnosed cases there are, and yet we know this is something that is not very practical as a process. But if COVID-19 was very contagious, the central issue is, people want to be free to live their lives, and that is, the aspect that counts. It is not just avoiding people from dying from the COVID-19 virus. It is that people would like to be free so they can live their lives and can prosper according to their views of how to best live their life without being restrained because of the COVID-19 virus.

Amukusana Bertha Nkandu, 42, housemaid; Lusaka, Zambia

Such as most people, I do not believe that it is COVID-19 in Zambia. How our government and public health services are asking people to fight a widespread pandemic when there is no COVID-19 infection to fight. People on social media and video platforms have been saying that SARS-Cov-2 is an ancient virus as today, and the novelty has dissipated. So even if this infection is here, it just one or two confirmed cases, and people still do not believe that it can cause deaths because of being infected. People of I know including myself and close relatives have never followed these false health regulations and guidelines on Coronavirus. These public health regulations and guidelines of social distancing, masking up, washing hands with soap, and avoiding handshakes or any form of body contact are true bogus, and people are not falling with that kind of foolishness. Our government and public health specialists are busy trotting's in the campaign with a crowd of unmasked people around them without social distancing, and they are asking the population to follow the health recommendation? Who can believe the falsity of Covid 19 with all that? And in fact, my pastor alongside a friend of mine who is a traditional healer, last week told us that our religion, strong genes, alcohol, and the tropical climate protect us from contracting the COVID-19 virus. Therefore, I am immune and continue to live my life at the fullest as everyone here. COVID-19 is a myth and a huge fake lie.

Esther Roseline Emmanuel, 29, esthetician; Pieton-Ville, Haiti

I heard that COVID-19 does not exist, and I do not follow these fake health restrictions, including wearing a face mask or social distancing at all. Also, my friend told me that if you go to the hospital even with a slight fever, they give a deadly injection to raise the number of deaths related to the pandemic to receive more international relief funding. So, my family and I would rather die at home than go to the hospital. All this is just about an outbreak of fever touching a larger part of the population, as usual, but not a COVID-19 virus. Again COVID-19 does not exist and that if we rely on Jesus Christ, we have nothing to worry about.

Seydou Lacina Moussa, 58, science teacher; Yamoussoukro, Ivory Coast.

Although exceptional times call for exceptional actions, but authorities should not maintain these types of measures indefinitely. People are not disposed to endure enormous disruptions to their everyday lives since they do not know when the disruptions will end and believe that authorities have been lying about COVID-19 just to get international relief funding. COVID-19 does not seem to be an enormous risk, especial-

ly here in Yamoussoukro where hot weather is often fatal to respiratory viruses, like COVID-19 virus. And in the nearly few months, the authorities asserted that the virus has been spreading here in the country (Ivory Coast), why the number of confirmed cases is still very low compared to other countries? Therefore, I do not see why people have to abide by their restricted recommendations, including staying home orders. People will not be following these recommendations as the disease is not here, it is just a pure fabrication from our authorities. Also, the mainstream media working for the authorities are trying to scare people and control our fears. The excellent news is that most people are at a very low risk of being infected with COVID-19 and then dying from it. COVID-19 is expected, like most outbreaks, to mount and fall in weeks or months and so is doubtful to kill that many people ever.

Abasiola Abiola Odjon, 45, self-employed working in the informal sector; Lagos, Nigeria.

The COVID-19 is a total myth and phony history set up by our greedy leaders for their profits. This COVID-19 looks like the others I heard in the past about EBOLA, HIV/AIDS, SARS, and about the swine flu alongside other outbreaks of viruses that have taken place in the country. But none of them led to anything catastrophic and do not justify such restricted measures such as a lockdown. I believe the factual truth is not being told to people, and people will not follow these fake authorities and health measures. Although, if this fake COVID-19 virus exists, every individual that will be infected or dies with that will be a misfortune for their family. But that is also true for car crashes, cancer, murder, and all premature deaths. So why authorities have been showing more concern about this fake COVID-19 virus when before they did not care about people suffering and poor living conditions. Incidentally, people died despite vaccination, proper medication, and a certain immunity. People should live life normally. Yes, washing the hands more often is fine. At least I conclude that COVID-19 it is mostly a normal flu pandemic. And I am a huge believer in living life entirely and not playing it safe all the time. In other words, the share of the pleasure contrasted with the risk is so enormous, I opt for the joy. Everything you do there is a risk, there is a probability that I will die one day, but I do not want to play it safe and not enjoying my life fully. So that is my attitude with the COVID-19 virus.

Mwimbi Cyrile Floribert, 28, climate change and ecological activist; Kinshasa, the Democratic Republic of the Congo.

I ponder if COVID-19 is attempting to tell the world something bigger. People have all been cautioned for years bout climate change and global warming. The existing world population is nearly 7.5 billion, and in fact, more than the globe can sustain. The population has been increasing at a fast pace, and people could gain from an urgent decrease in the worldwide population by less than 2-3 billion of the least useful inhabitants. And our least most productive inhabitants are the aging and retired people that the COVID-19 affects hardest. Allowing the disease to run its normal courses could be a long-term blessing to upcoming generations of human beings. The outcome would be a huge decrease in the aging population, which statistically absorbs the greater part of the medical resources in the last few years of their life. It also should decrease the lower intelligence quotient (IQ) population, which was foolish enough to not prevent gatherings or wash their hands along with all that. So, as I am concerned, COVID-19 is a long-term blessing for me as it will help to decrease the overpopulated planet.

Ousmane Faye Diop, 48, an economist; Ziguinchor, Dakar, Senegal

What has occurred with this COVID-19 is completely ridiculous and crazy. This fake disease is disturbing the entire world economy. People are looking into the eyes of a dangerous Great Depression that will overthrow our fragile governments, all because of an overreaction and hyping of this fake virus. Far more people die of the flu, Ebola, HIV/AIDS, Malaria, and even smoking than this bogus virus. Governments should not shut down commerce and impose foolish strict orders because of such diseases. Perhaps it results from absolute idiots who just think about halting a disease that has a lower death rate than the general flu virus. Either way, this country is eyeing at significant economic implications for their ways of battling a bogus infection that has resulted in the economic policy of burned earth.

Jerry Fritz Pissarro, 38, financial analyst; St Thomas, U.S. Virgin Island (USVI)

Many people are asking why this COVID-19 has been stirred up into a major fear when the yearly flu kills far more people. Perhaps they have enlisted the conspiracy contingents from in a foreign country who transform everything into the end of the world and are so enthusiastic to paint death and misery as a deadly weapon for mass financial devastation. They do not understand that they are being played for idiots, spitting out many conspiracies such as biological weapons laced with AIDS that will kill half of the population without a single piece of evidence. This is precisely how government and health care specialists provoke mass fear, through falsehoods, deception, and manipulating people's ignorance. It is how they persuade people they are all going to die because COVID-19 is deadly when it is unfounded.

The continued lockdowns are unjustified and useless in preventing deaths from COVID-19. Today the COVID-19-panic gives government and healthcare specialist fuel and cover for its attacks on freedom and poses a question the government does not want to reply: If freedom can be taken away in periods of disaster? The government has no power to impose how many people decide on a social gathering or have a social drink with friends and relatives. People have far more to worry about this Government dictatorship than people do from the COVID-19 virus. People's liberty is natural and personal, and they cannot sacrifice it for the bogus COVID-19 pandemic. Canceling public events is completely ridiculous, and there is no logical justification for it.

Alima Asma Assana, 33, analyst; Bobo Dioulasso, Burkina Faso

As far I am concerned this COVID-19 is fake and it has not disturbed me at all, I still can go to a bar and have a drink and kick it with all my girlfriends. People believe all these so-called restrictions are boring and unproductive for our life. My girlfriends and I are not scared of the COVID-19 virus since we believe it is having been exag-

gerated by the government and the media when it should not be. I even do not wear a face mask either inside my work office or outside in the street because I did not feel like it. The authorities should loosen these restrictions and let people decide how to leave their lives. If I get it, I get it, but the authorities and COVID-19 will not have to dictate to me how to live my life fully. People are tired of it and should be in charge of their actions. Our so-called leaders need to stop being monarchs and blindly following everything coming from in foreign countries, instead, they should work harder to decrease the significant gap in poverty that poor people face daily.

Mboma, Mbonghe Nkono, 62, retired science teacher; Bafoussam, Cameroon

Although the government imposed their restrictions such as stay home order, I have been traveling across the country to different cities either to visit my relatives and friends or to enjoy my retirement time, even though it is not suggested. A friend of mine who is a nurse in Yaoundé informed me that the sooner I will get infected with the virus, the faster my body system will be protected. Therefore, by traveling across cities, I hope to get the virus and provide my body with a stronger immune system. I just want to get it over with, since I do not still believe COVID-19 is that bad, even people can be asymptomatic and bring it back to their own families. My cousin mentioned to me he has been exposed to the virus because someone in his workplace was sick with some undiagnosed sickness and now it turns out to be COVID-19, and therefore he believes to be fine, considering that he should be immune by now. So, I am enjoying my life unafraid and hoping others will do the same, as government restrictions and COVID-19 would not prevent me to be joyful and fearless at all. I am a retired person who gave too much to this country and has little time to live as today, so I am enjoying, and nobody could tell otherwise. Spending time with friends and eating wonderful food with a nice cold drink at any bar or nightclub is more valued that COVID-19, which may not be present at all.

CHAPTER FIVE

What next? Will the World be Normal Again?

It has been over a year that the planet has survived this new deadly pathogen, and the world, especially Haiti and the nations of Africa, are nowhere close to the final stretches of this fight.

While most people hoped they had a reset switch that could make COVID-19 vanish and they could awaken from this nightmare realizing that it was only a dream, the reality is that a new normal must be established because there are mutations and variants of the virus yet to be identified and controlled. In most places people believe they will resume their everyday existence without concern for what may come next. The reality, however, is that as much as things may appear somewhat "normal" on the surface, many things have changed and may well continue to change. Until sufficient people are immunized to achieve population herd immunity, until all variants are identified and the lethality of each known, and effective vaccines to inhibit their spread and impact are created, COVID-19 will continue to lurk quietly in the background of our everyday lives.

The other stark reality is that the virus is now here, and it will stay. It will evolve, mutate, and remain in the earth. Whether there will be periods of dormancy when infections are minimal to almost non-existent, or whether it will continue to spread throughout segments of the population as those unvaccinated or having immunocompromised systems, or pre-existing and comorbid illnesses and the elderly succumb to it, none of these are known factors at this time. The truth is that pandemics have occurred in the past and will occur again. The virulence of them cannot be predicted, which means the greatest weapons we have are the facts and knowledge we learn and apply from this one.

Soumya Swaminathan, a chief scientist for the World Health Organization (WHO), has stated "We know this virus is not going away soon. It's established itself and will keep on transmitting wherever it's able to do so," and "We know we must live with this."[203]

Dr. Fauci, the Director of the National Institute of Allergy and Infectious Diseases (NIAID) and the United States' leading health expert, and one of the world's most trusted voices on all things COVID-19-associated, concurred with this assertion, stating: "There is an increasing sign that the novel coronavirus could turn out to be a cyclical (seasonal) infection, similar to colds and the flu." He added that "What we are perceiving now in the Southern Hemisphere and southern African countries is that we are having cases appearing as they go into their winter season. If, in fact, they have a substantial outbreak, it will be inevitable, therefore, we need to be prepared for the next cycle."[204]

Mohammad Sajadi, a professor at the University of Maryland's Institute of Human Virology, said "the hypothesis that this virus exhibits a seasonality is based in part on the behavior of other respiratory viruses in temperate climates, as well as the lack of major covid-19 outbreaks in countries south of China, where travel patterns suggested the potential for large-scale spread."[205, 206]

In a study on the effects of weather and COVID-19, researchers Shaman, Goldman, and Lipsitch, quote David Heymann, a professor at the London School of Hygiene and Tropical Medicine, as having stated "there are two main reasons the coronavirus could exhibit some seasonality. One has more to do with human behavior because people tend not to be in confined spaces for extended periods during the summer. This could somewhat hinder the spread of the virus. The other reason, which is more of an unknown right now, has to do with the virus itself, specifically its transmissibility in different seasons."[207, 208]

Devi Sridhar, chair of Global Public Health at the University of Edinburgh, has also implied that the spread COVID-19 may slow down in the warmer months, compared to influenza, which usually spreads from November to April or May, but will not disappear as many people may believe. Sridhar stated that "Over the past decade there has been an increasing number of viruses and bacterial infections spilling over into humans and as long as we have close contact between animals and humans, we will continue to have spillover events. And we see that through urbanization, deforestation, and having wet markets. The virus will still spread even after a successful vaccine is broadly offered because of those people who will prefer not to get vaccinated and will live with the virus for a while."[210]

Hillary Godwin, dean of the University of Washington's School of Public Health, in sync with the points of view of other experts asserted that, "A year from now, and even beyond that, we should expect to still see people wearing masks in public, especially those who are more vulnerable to COVID-19 and that the big part of the future will be greater expectations around masks." She added that "Mask-wearing will become more normal, the way it has been in many Asian countries in recent years, and we will see a shift toward that."[211]

However, none of the mitigation and prevention measures will be effective, nor will there be simple solutions. We will need tough discipline from all people for the mandates and protections to work. It will require people to collaborate and work cooperatively as they have never done before.

As health specialists are still learning about COVID-19, it has also placed a focus on the disparities within healthcare systems around the world, especially in Africa, Haiti, and the USVI and the difficulties linked with viewing health policies in isolation from social aspects.

This is the time for the health world to promote systems

that value prevention and recognize that all policies are health policies because all policies - economic, transportation, city planning designs, etc. all have effects upon health, be it physical or mental health. Governments and public health policymakers should make certain they address all aspects that can deliver and sustain health, not just trying to support people once they are in poor health.

There needs to be a sense of balance between preventive and curative approaches, unbiased access to social services, policy guidelines that highlight the social determinants of health, and a move away from illness care/curative systems that are now operating. Diagnosing and treating people after they become ill is unavoidable but making prevention the primary focus allows for early mitigation of disease and helps to reduce disease burden. This is an approach which has been argued to be costly up front due to the prices attached to screening methodologies and equipment such as MRIs, CT scans, etc., but curative treatment is far more expensive over the long haul. With the curative aspect, it is challenging to have a population that is well, because this approach focuses on the disease in the person, rather than centering on social factors and proximate elements that affect and cause disease. Prevention is the proper panacea. Governments and populations must collaborate to prevent disease transmission from the outset.

The current vaccines for COVID-19 have been developed from the prevention approach - as most vaccines are created.

Studying the virus and treating it from the knowledge base we now have places the world in a position to not only develop better more effective vaccines with greater efficacy, but also to craft more effective behavioral guidelines to minimize the chances of contracting the virus all together.

Among the recommendations imposed as the safest routes to halt the transmission of COVID-19 were to stay home whenever that could be done and wash hands often. While these appeared like suitable recommendations, in Haiti and Africa this was not always possible because of lack of access to hygienic sanitation and clean water.

In Haiti there are entire communities and towns, and in Africa, cities, and countries, where one must walk miles to access fresh, clean water. If washing one's hands is one of the simplest and most efficient means of preventing the spread of disease (which it has been proven to be), then governments and public health officials need to address remediation of this barrier not only for the health of their populations, but also for the sake of their country's financial survival because caring for the ill is costly. The old adage holds true: an ounce of prevention is better than a pound of cure.

During the COVID-19 pandemic and in the aftermath of other natural disasters, communities have been placed on boil water orders to ensure water is clean. This temporary stop-gap measure works well if one has ready access water; but when water is not available and the purchase of hand sanitizer is also not an option, how do people avoid disease? Thus, improved housing and water infrastructure are essential needed improvements the governments of African nations and Haiti must consider not only in light of the effects and impacts of COVID-19, but for any other pandemic or epidemic that may arise in the future.

Whenever health, housing systems, and economic systėms are in shambles, there is no more opportune time and opportunity to reconstruct from the ground up. As the major portion of gross domestic product (GDP) of many of these countries is devoted to areas other than the health care systems, reallocation of funds to those policy fields focused on improving the social determinants of health will require significant realignment.

In response to COVID-19, all these areas declared a state of emergency and their governments invoked the use of emergency laws. This was the perfect time for them to also broaden the definition of medically necessary services within the emergency laws and pass comprehensive health improvement measures, such as national health programs. They need to create health policies that are all-inclusive and consider the bidirectional correlation between preventive and curative measures, which should be analyzed within the societal framework of existing determinants of health including gender, race, education, and socioeconomic aspects.

Such an approach, coupled with integrative policies over-reactive measures, public programs over privatization, and the adoption of preventive measures to prevent sickness, melded with collaboration and partnership with governments that have successfully improved health systems, would help Haiti and African nations bring their health systems and public health services into the 21st century. These countries should seize the opportunity for partnerships across countries and among governments, private sectors, and community organizations for benefits of overall improvement and proper system expansion.

Africa, the USVI, and Haiti Need Better COVID-19 Strategies.

Despite the introduction of vaccines, new and more viral variants of the virus are bringing exhaustion and new cases to Haiti and the many countries of Africa.

No one can predict when an epidemic or pandemic of another novel virus may occur causing a significant contamination necessitating intensive hospital care or may contribute to mass mortalities. Management of the response by relying on inpatient beds and access to ventilators at broken hospitals as preventive health mandates are relaxed will be an ineffective approach with the hope for a practical result. Improvement of health infrastructure, funding and acquisition of equipment, personnel trained to maintain and repair equipment, hiring competent staff and providers, making health a priority for all citizens, these are the things that will help combat the next epidemic or pandemic.

The COVID-19 virus has been fatal to the elderly, but evidence emerged over the course of the pandemic showing that younger healthy people between the ages of 20 and 54 were being taken ill and dying according to a report from the Centers for Disease Control and Prevention (CDC).[212] While many believed this segment of the population was immune to the virus, the CDC data showed otherwise. However, the data may not have been quite descriptive of what was taking place in many African countries as the accuracy of data collection and reporting from the continent is questionable and not reliable.[213] It also may not have been an accurate reflection of the virus's run in Africa or Haiti because the CDC report was based on a review of the first 2,500 registered cases in the United States of America, as it was expected the earliest surge of cases would be the harshest because of testing limitations at the time.[214]

It is possible that many African countries and Haiti may see more cases of younger persons suffering, especially if the virus continues to mutate to more virulent strains and because the predominant population of these areas happens to be non-elderly.

If the mutated strains continue to thrive, and restrictions and preventive measures are loosened, it is entirely possible that Haiti and nations within Africa could experience surges in cases. Such a scenario would be strenuous upon these areas and their already weak health infrastructure. It is imperative that the lessons learned from this first round of the pandemic be followed up with stringent policies and plans for both response and recovery as the choice between healthy economies and healthy populations is a fallacious dichotomy, as these areas cannot have one without the other.

Seeking the help and guidance of other nations which have been successful in halting large scale viral transmission and reopening their economies, will be invaluable not only if the variants prove prolific, but just as importantly for preparation for future epidemics and pandemics.

Haiti and Africa must legislate containment strategies formed in the interest of public health and epidemiology that define how each will conscientiously remain open while sustaining or reducing the rates of the novel coronavirus disease among their populations.

The capacity of the virus to burgeon at a rapid pace suggests that by the time the seriousness of the situation is accepted, it could well be too late.

To successfully remain open, it will be necessary to enact practical and basic steps, such as restraining the number of people at social gatherings, addressing capacity at public businesses, and issuing workplace safety standards. Measures such as these, will help keep economies thriving, thereby reducing the economic and psychological impacts brought about by more stern measures such as total lockdowns and confinement. Even now, as cases are in a downward trend, it is still important to wear face masks as one never knows if someone they encounter has been exposed to a variant, or if they have not been vaccinated. This single protective measure is one that can, in fact, help save lives and minimize transmission as data has repeatedly revealed that it is one of the most efficient and easy approaches to curb the spread of COVID-19. While not always comfortable or convenient, the reality is that wearing a face mask or cloth face coverings protects the individual, their relatives, friends, and the communities at large.

Politics and political ideology or affiliation should not be factors in the creation and implementation of measures to protect people. Authorities and government leadership should do all they can to strengthen the capacity of all communities and cities to protect their citizens and residents regardless of social class, status, or political stance.

Definitive instruction and leadership should be provided to local and community level government alongside enforcement resources should local leaders decide to formulate more strict mandates when the national authorities are reluctant to do so.

What Happened During COVID-19, and What May be Coming

COVID-19 changed almost every facet of life around the globe in a year-and-a-half. While evidence credits Africa and Haiti with responding right away by implementing widespread lockdowns to slow the spread of COVID-19, such approaches came with enormous costs medically, economically, socially, and psychologically, and they were not always kept in place for sufficient periods of time to thwart the spread of disease.

Critical health care services were disturbed, including infant vaccination, cancer screening, and HIV treatment programs, and other necessary medical services and treatment operations with far-reaching and severe consequences.[215, 216]

From another point of view, where lockdowns were lifted too quickly, transmission reemerged, forcing some countries to re-close businesses. Though it was normal for governments to react to impractical circumstances by centering on the problems, their remediation of reopening left the populations with puzzling messages about the continued risks of this infectious virus. Efforts at innovative methods to fight COVID-19 have not worked out as projected. Questions about balancing the public interest with civil liberties to issues around using anti-malarial drugs that were later found ineffective, all had inherent weaknesses and were believed to be mistakes on the part of the public health emergency response.

Governments around the world perceived their overall COVID-19 responses were a strategy of balancing approaches to assess public health with economic health, and they asserted that a balance could be struck by pointing out the low death rates in other countries compared to their own. But this thinking was challenged by evidence coupled with expert points of view, which demonstrated that the balancing strategies were misguided because they could not achieve economic health until there was public health. Also, most people believed COVID-19 responses were framed inaccurately from the beginning, deploring the hyper-debated climate around wearing masks, social distancing mandates, travel bans, and economic closures. People were concerned that in their approaches, governments had not accurately balanced medical advice in the decision-making on a range of issues, whether it was to re-open the economy or the unwillingness to enforce nationwide wearing of face masks, social distancing, and travel restrictions. It did not help the confidence of citizens that some countries passed several key decisions without the acknowledgment of renowned scientists' points of view.

One measure that met stark failure even though it received some citizen support was the eagerness by some governments to mandate the use of anti-malarial drugs against concerns expressed by a multitude of health professionals. Since making their social media debut, hydroxychloroquine and chloroquine have turned out to be contentious issues in contradictory COVID-19 pandemic debates.

Varying views on the efficacy of these malarial drugs, ranging from magic cure to harmful treatments, were bandied about in the public arena. The debate served as a dividing line in many countries, with government sympathizers and friendly media channels echoing their passions for the use of the drugs, while most of the population and many health specialists insisted there were no consistent data or science showing the two drugs could help cure or even be an effective treatment for COVID-19 symptoms.

While health specialists' views on the drugs were far from unanimous and cautioned officials against using the unverified drugs, there were those nations that felt confident in moving forward with granting permission to administer the two drugs. For instance, Nigeria's National Agency for Food and Drug Administration and Control (NAFDAC) confirmed the use of chloroquine to treat COVID-19. NAFDAC Director-General, Professor Christianah Mojisola Adeyeye, insisted that chloroquine could be used in the early stages of the COVID-19 infection as a prophylactic treatment. She further lent substantiation to the use of chloroquine stating, "the director-general of Senegal's drug regulatory body, who is also the director-general of the regional regulatory body, ordered chloroquine from a company in Ota, Ogun State and distributed it to 15 member-countries," adding, "if something is effective prophylactically, it means that the disease will not progress."[217]

Although some countries endorsed the use of the divisive anti-malarial drug hydroxychloroquine, most, especially hospitals, made decisions not to dispense chloroquine and hydroxychloroquine as a form of COVID-19 treatment. The WHO declared that it would stop the use of hydroxychloroquine as part of its global solidarity trial amid a safety review.[218]

The United States Food and Drug Administration (FDA) also cautioned against using hydroxychloroquine outside of a hospital or in clinical trial settings.[219] The French government and several other developed countries banned the use of the drugs as treatment for COVID-19.[220] The determination to ban the use of hydroxychloroquine and chloroquine occurred after interim trial results revealed that the anti-malaria drugs had limited or no change in numbers of deaths of patients hospitalized for COVID-19.

The tragedy that unfolded throughout the globe was that as governments and public health specialists fought over what was valid scientific information that should be followed and what was conjecture, the numbers of cases and the deaths continued to rise daily.

People hoped their leaders would change their approaches, learn from mistakes made, and rely more on medical knowledge as they continued to debate and make decisions. But authorities argued that the determinations made were done with public health experts at the forefront, balancing those with a need to avoid devastating impacts on the economies.

There were, however, scientists who claimed some authorities did not receive the evidence presented either because they had been advised by other scientists who themselves, did not believe the evidence, or who had political ambitions and thus chose to be in alignment with the government position.

Scientists standing on behalf of the suffering populations alleged that government representatives did not attempt their best, and the decisions formulated into policy were not based on all-inclusive approaches. Yet, it has been speculated that one of the things Africa, Haiti and the USVI did, which may have saved them from the reality of the catastrophic losses predicted at the start of the pandemic, is that they closed their borders, severely restricting travel into and out of the countries. This quick action is credited for the numbers of COVID victims and cases being far less than were predicted for these areas.

Another factor that may have played a significant role in the virus transmission and lethality is the population structure of most African countries and Haiti: the population pyramids are mid-to bottom heavy indicating the primary population is young. COVID-19 has been repeatedly shown to have greater transmissibility among the elderly and those over 60, than the young. A good example of this population difference is demonstrated by the fact that Niger's population is 25 times younger than that of the United Kingdom.[221] South Africa had the highest numbers of cases and rates of death in Africa in the height of the pandemic, yet its death rate was still "only 40% that of the United Kingdom."[222] So, even with high numbers, Africa still has not experienced the catastrophic outcomes predicted and projected by scientists and public health specialists around the world.

It would seem that speculations about the impact of the virus in Africa and Haiti not having been fulfilled as projected would mean all was well for these areas during the height of the pandemic; however, that is not the case. Leadership's messaging about different localities or regions which recorded surges in cases and presented high threat levels were deficient and confusing and should have been phased to facilitate detection of the results because of the gap between behavior and cases as this may have avoided surges in concentrated areas.

On a worldwide scale, the African continent by mid-June 2021 reported 5.4 million cases with 140,000 deaths, demonstrating that although case numbers had continued to increase, the death toll was still small considering the number of cases and the total population of the vast continent. The USVI reported 3,385 cases with 30 deaths in the same time period; while Haiti reported only 17,902 cases and 398 deaths.[223-225] Although these numbers paint a grand picture of the COVID-19 response, the fact is that the transmission rates and virulence of the variants are not yet known and the advent of these into the African continent, Haiti, and the USVI could prove to be more than their understaffed, inadequately equipped, and failing health systems and infrastructure can handle. As this work went to publication, it was reported that the number of cases across Africa had surged to 6 million with 156,000 deaths.[226]

It is believed the new mutation is more highly transmissible than COVID-19. Recent information reported by the BBC as of May 2021, reveals that the new variants, although they appear to be spreading and accounting for a surge in cases in 20 African nations, cannot be "easily tracked because the testing required to identify them isn't widely available." [227] This means that, at the present time, information about the Delta variant is speculative. This variant, first reported in Africa in Uganda, is now present in Kenya, Morocco, Algeria, South Africa, Botswana, Angola, DR Congo, Nigeria, Zambia, and Zimbabwe, with South Africa having the greatest numbers of cases.[228] Nigeria reported that a new variant has been discovered in that country, but details as to whether it is the same Delta variant or a different strain, remains to be revealed.[229] The African Centers for Disease Control sanctioned the creation of a broader network of laboratories to help the continent better identify variants of the virus more speedily.

Though no one could predict the trajectory of the virus in the African continent, Haiti, or the USVI, if the current trends in the transmission of the present identified variants changes, the health care systems, including hospitals, could well be exhausted and the conditions under which health care providers work could become far harsher and demanding.

Current measures to reopen economies while still encouraging preventive behaviors has caused some confusion and puzzlement as nation-wide mask mandates have been rescinded in some localities but not in others as economies struggle to fully reopen.

More confusion also exists around what is safe in terms of mask wearing and what is not. Some officials say if one is fully vaccinated there is no need to where masks; while others say there is not yet sufficient evidence of the longevity of the vaccines or if one can still incur the virus even after vaccination. In fact, at the completion of the writing of this book it was reported that almost 6,000 fully vaccinated persons had been diagnosed with COVID-19.[230, 231] This fact, more than any other: that those fully vaccinated can in fact, still get the virus, supports the need for governments to exercise caution in lifting mandates for masks and maybe even slow down and more closely monitor the reopening of businesses. Facing up to this fact, putting it in the public arena in a big way, would send a strong and vital message to populations about their need to remain safe and prevent transmission.

In the beginning, it appeared that African nations were doing all they could to speedily address the encroaching pandemic. The first case was reported February 14, 2020, and within weeks – by March 4th, Nigeria had completed sequencing of the SARS CoV-2 (virus that causes COVID -19) genome.[232] In South Africa, testing was ramped up to identify existing cases quickly. In October 2020, it was reported that African nations were going to roll out COVID-19 Rapid Testing which was predicted to expand efforts to test greater numbers of people.[233] It was believed this would help in not only providing more expansive testing, but true numbers in reporting would be more readily available because with insufficient testing thousands, possibly millions of cases, were being missed.[234]

Prior to mid-2020, doubts were expressed as to testing effectiveness in the continent, although lab representatives of many of the nations backed their testing reliability, denouncing what they considered unnecessary inquiry. There was a broad unanimity, however, among the population and many of those in charge of health policies that testing effectiveness was highly questionable and testing rates were meaningless, which contributed to misrepresenting officials' knowledge of the extent to which COVID-19 had travelled through the population. When the pandemic began, in the entire continent there were only two laboratories that could analyze COVID-19 test results which leant some credence to the doubts circulating as to the veracity of results being reported and the capability of the labs to properly analyze and report testing results. By October 2020, instead of just two labs on the continent, there were 750, and it was believed this increase in lab capacity combined with the roll out of rapid testing would improve testing all around and result in better identification of hotspots.[235]

Cost was another impediment to rolling out widespread testing. Reagents to conduct the COVID-19 tests were expensive, and with the demand being world-side, African countries found it difficult to compete financially. This had a double negative effect in that not only were insufficient numbers of people being tested to better identify where virus pockets were, but some nations began picking and choosing whom would be tested leaving the poor in fear of dying from the dreaded virus.[236]

In Nigeria, the continent's most heavily populated country of 200 million and one of the wealthiest, the capacity to run COVID-19 tests sat at a paltry 2500 a day. And although during the last few months of 2020 improvements had been implemented, Nigeria still had tested 11 times fewer people than Brazil – a nation with similar population size and public health challenges. This is also in stark contrast to New York City, with a population of 8.4 million, where upwards of 20,000 tests per day were being conducted.[237-239] Further, on its own continent, Nigeria compared poorly to South Africa where that country had performed about 10 tests per 1,000, while Nigeria had only conducted 0.23 tests per 1,000.[239]

Other African nations have had their share of difficulties, false reporting, errors, and insufficiency of equipment and trained staff. The health minister of Tanzania "suspended the head of the East African country's national laboratory after the lab sent back positive COVID-19 test results for samples taken from a goat, a quail, and pawpaw."[240] Speaking during a televised oath ceremony for a new cabinet minister, Tanzanian President John Magufuli, claimed he "suspected a dirty game was being played at the lab."[241] It was further reported that during discussions about importing test kits, the Prime Minister warned that "Tanzanians should not view every piece of assistance from abroad as good for this nation." He also advised other countries in Africa using comparable kits to perform tests of their own, predicting they would corroborate the findings in Tanzania."

Along with not having enough testing equipment, the initial problems with labs, and general underreporting was the problem of reaching those living in rural areas.

Many in sparsely populated regions of the continent resisted being tested because of beliefs that the virus was a hoax or that the testing could, itself, cause the virus, or that the medicine and potions of juju or local healers was sufficient to save them. These groups were not being tested.

Dr. Matshidiso Moeti, WHO Regional Director for Africa, recognized the lack of testing was "leading to some under-reporting of COVID-19 cases and preventing us from understanding the full picture of the COVID-19 pandemic in Africa."[242]

The populations of many African nations, Haiti, the USVI, and indeed around the world, have shared similar experiences and emotions during the pandemic: sorrow, denial, anger, bargaining, and even depression. But moving from each of these to acceptance is a critical factor in our progressing beyond the disease dictating our lives and livelihoods and our taking control given the fact that COVID-19 is here to stay. This change in framing may appear challenging, but it is crucial as energy centered on debating about problems is energy not used on improving and achieving results.

Undeniably, defining challenges can be an essential initial step in identifying solutions.

However, when it involves the discussion of wider policies, leaders of these governments should be cautious not to get trapped at the challenge-discovering stage.

As these countries pursue efforts to implement needed solutions, there are four principles leaders should apply to guide their approaches.

1- Be Specific

Leaders should work to change the public debate from the general to the specific, obliging the populations and themselves out of the proverbial weeds.

Much of the discussion surrounding lockdowns, social distancing, and the wearing of masks, for instance, has functioned at an uncooperative level of generalization. Policies of this scale have wide-reaching impacts on medical, economic, legal, and social factors. Many policies were not applied evenly, disproportionately affecting various geographic regions and different employment sectors (formal and informal).

Leaders cannot (and should not) assess the suitability of policies in confinement without defining options. The value of several exit strategies, along with reporting what they entail and their specificity, is lost on the population for whom they are designed when proffered without efforts to suggest workable alternatives along with searching for proactive approaches. When leaders adamantly demand enforcement of such mandates or substitute harsher restrictions, they place their populations in a deplorable level of threat.

The debate on reopening schools was a great example of governments and other leaders not evaluating the breath of considerations necessary to ensure the safety of students and faculty. The insistence upon only two alternatives in the absence of fully understanding or examining the ramifications of both, has led to disastrous consequences for students. The alternatives given were (1) to close schools entirely, thereby forcing all students to continue their education in a home environment with professional assistance available only via virtual platforms for specified amounts of time during the day; and (2) to attend school with everyone social distancing and wearing masks and face-shields.

Some of the issues inherent in each of these choices were:

- Many in-home environments were not conducive to sustaining and managing learning as parents who were not teachers or educators had jobs themselves, and thus could not engage in direct supervision and assistance, often leaving children to fend for themselves while teachers attempted, virtually, to hold order and teach the days' lesson.
- Those parents who were teachers, had to teach their classes while trying to keep an eye on the child-students in their own homes.
- Children with learning disabilities and challenges found themselves floundering as the support systems usually provided during the school day were no longer available or did not work as well in a virtual environment.
- The development of key psychological and social skills was basically put on hold: Socialization skills of younger children were delayed as their engagement with others of their ages were stymied by pandemic mandates to remain indoors and forced the closure of day care centers and elementary schools. High schoolers were bereft of critical relationship forming opportunities with peers as they were reduced to only internet and phone interactions which foster a false sense of relationship in the absence of real physical communication. In college, budding young

adults transitioning from their teens, develop higher level skills of professionalism, networking, tolerance of broader diversity, and sometimes form life-long friendships. These opportunities for growth were all stymied by rules and strategies formulated in the face of the pandemic.

- For those parents and educators who moved forward with in-school presence, achieving social distancing of at least 6 feet between persons front, back, and sides, meant cutting the number of students who could be in a classroom. In places such as the United States, this could mean a classroom of 30 students being cut down to half that size, and rotations of students twice a day to accommodate all 30. In many African countries where some classrooms have as many as 56 students, and buildings are smaller, enforcement of social distancing was difficult to achieve forcing learning to be conducted outdoors, and in most cases, the complete closure of schools.
- Closure of schools has led to many students falling behind in their grade level as learning in a virtual environment is exceptionally different from in-class. Those students who are kinesthetic learners, students requiring additional physical support and tutoring, those whose motivation is spurred by being around others in a learning environment, have all incurred

categorical challenges in trying to maintain attention on studies in this new world.

- In some countries schools did not have a budget to accommodate the additional expense of purchasing masks and face shields. Impoverished families unable to afford even the most inexpensive masks due to loss of work and the accompanying meager income, found themselves unable to send their children to school even when schools were reopened.

Leaders did not ask the pertinent questions at the outset of the pandemic. Instead, many waited until the pandemic had a strangle hold on the population, and panic about what to do and how to do it had set in before they were available to ask pertinent questions and conduct solid research into viable, feasible, pragmatic, applicable answers. What does social distancing for all schools look like? Are there differences in building structure and size that will affect the ability to social distance? Can some instruction be shifted outside? How can indoor events be organized further without harm? The action of establishing alternatives is instructive as it provides the population something tangible to debate.

In analyzing, specifics approaches should not only have been about decreasing COVID-19 transmission and death, but also should have focused on the reduction of wider impacts of the pandemic. In some of these countries, schools offer many essential services to different communities, for instance, not only schooling but also meal programs, especially for less fortunate children. Careful consideration should have been directed to the continuity of such programs in the pandemic environment.

Healthcare services suffered incredible impacts with disruptions of regular medical care such as cancer screening and child immunizations. The delivery of care also changed as people were reluctant to visit health care facilities for worry of infection, with many therefore choosing decentralized care at remote offices, or even home-based care.

By breaking diffuse larger problems into specific smaller ones, an outwardly intractable problem comes to be more workable.

2- Compare Worldwide

Researching and reviewing best practices from around the world would be helpful to nations struggling to address disease proliferation, especially when they are attacking the same health and medical issues such as a pandemic causing virus or disease.

This produces a wealth of information from which alternative approaches may be gleaned and learned. For instance, what can be learned from the enormous testing campaigns carried out in China, or the clear crisis communication that was carried out in New Zealand? After the 2015 Middle East Respiratory Syndrome (MERS) pandemic, South Korea enhanced its early detection monitoring systems and infection prevention protocols. In Japan, the emphasis was on decreasing close-range human interaction at various crowd venues and centering detection of large infection clusters using several groups of public health nurses. Reliable hotlines and apps in Vietnam kept the population up to date on the most recent information.

On the internet site "Our World in Data", authorities and public health specialists can review examples in worldwide health to learn from South Korea, Vietnam, and Germany regarding their effective COVID-19 responses.

The UK's Royal Society of Scientists unveiled the DELVE (Data Evaluation and Learning for Viral Epidemics) initiative, whereby multidisciplinary groups collect evidence from other countries and synthesize these into comprehensive reports and policy suggestions and review commonalities in methodologies for tracing, isolating, and testing contrasted policies across nations. They emphasized the short turnaround times of testing results and the use of apps to improve manual tracing by performing automated follow-up symptom checks.

The fact is, there is much to be gleaned and applied to policy and approach from nations around the globe. Africa, Haiti, and the USVI should research these, make note of them, learn from them, and apply those that are best suited to their countries and populations.

3- Think nationwide

Once leaders and stakeholders have highlighted best practices and approaches the next step is policy inclusion and implementation. Grave consideration and in-depth evaluation of how to effectively roll out new public health measures in rural and remote areas must be undertaken if pandemics or local epidemics are to be effectively controlled.

Such control may be difficult to ensure in countries wherein large populations of immigrants reside as some may be undocumented, and thus unwilling to share information about their health status and contacts. These factors must be included in pandemic preparation and response plans. Public health programs must include language that addresses such fringe populations informing them of the dire consequences of the disease or virus and assuring them of safety when coming forth for help and treatment. It must be kept in mind that across-the-board solutions do not work in all scenarios or communities, and top-down approaches can falter when unforeseen difficulties arise in the enactment and enforcement of preventive health measures and rules.

Mathematical models can help gauge expectations and how quickly labs need to turn around test outcomes, the number of contacts that need to be traced, and how many need to be placed under isolation and quarantine. Some models may also be used to extrapolate, over a given course of time, some of the actions necessary to achieve desired outcomes.

To better tailor approaches for densely populated urban cities and rural areas where sanitation and water sources are compromised, authorities should also consider solutions from within

– i.e., those accomplishing the most effective work in the field.

Assessing the work and outcomes achieved by those working on the front lines, i.e. contact tracers, health care providers, and other essential workers, can yield knowledge that informs strategies best suited to given populations and areas. Those in the field have first-hand awareness of cultural and religious norms that may affect trust in medications, vaccines, regulations, and compliance with mandates. In addition, public health and government leaders should scour their nation to find out what innovations have been developed at the grass roots level to help stem the tide of disease transmission.

When representation from all areas of a nation and all socioeconomic levels are incorporated into the strategizing, solutions that are realistic and equitable can be developed and deployed to the betterment of all. This can motivate lasting change.

4- Build to Learn

A framework for learning, like a blueprint for collecting factual insights to inform evidence-based decisions, should be encouraged, and developed.

Over the previous year several online platforms such as the COVID Tracking Project, COVID Act Now, COVID Exit Strategy, and Johns Hopkins Testing Insights Initiative, and the WHO Coronavirus Disease (COVID-19) Dashboard, to list just a few, have risen to assist scientists in checking data. These reporting platforms allow national leaders and public health specialists to evaluate at a glance what is occurring worldwide, within their country, and to compare data against other potential data sources useful in projecting where diseases may impact, areas of high versus low infection, and demographics of those affected.

These platforms are usually data driven, receiving inputs from local epidemiologists, other public health specialists, and authorized government and private officials. By spotting the source of transmission, they will be able to generate reports showing the riskiness of diverse activities in given areas. For instance, although evidence has shown that scientists are able to connect the spread of viruses and diseases to gatherings at nightclubs, beaches, meetings, and churches, there remains some skepticism about movie theaters, subways, and airplanes.[243- 246]

Barun Mathema, Ph.D., an assistant professor of epidemiology at the Columbia University Mailman School of Public Health, said that churches and places of worship can "potentially fill a lot of the checkboxes" on the list of things that allow COVID-19 to easily spread.[247]

Finding beneficial ways forward is as much about determining low-risk areas as it is about finding high-risk ones. With businesses re-opening or implementing new mitigation measures, the landscape of settings is shifting. Governments and public health specialists need to make greater contributions in time and resources to gather and research complex tracing data to produce new and actionable insights so they can better understand disease progression and impacts as the lifestyles of the populations evolves. Potential cohort research, where populations are studied over a given period of time, can produce high-value data.

As new data gathering platforms are developed and tested, nations should begin planning for and determining what data sets will be most helpful and relevant for future epidemics and pandemics. This information will be based on what was already found to be most informative for decision making, and in reviewing challenges and problems incurred in the COVID-19 and other previous pandemics. These efforts can be rewarding overall as the outcomes may be more definitive and beneficial.

At the beginning of the pandemic, there was criticism "that clinical trials of various COVID-19 therapies were not being conducted fast enough, as the clinical research community was not prepared for the disruption caused by the COVID-19 pandemic, a force majeure that has impacted the operations and conduct of trials globally", therefore, treatment should be authorized based on limited data.[248] Yet, those who forged forward with randomized trials produced high-quality data that generated both successes and losses, "even several trial medications that were not allowed for any indication in any country were used outside of clinical experimentation protocols."[249]

Matthew P. et al. (2020) in their published article claimed that "there was a strong ethical and clinical argument for replacing such "random" care with randomized care, in which patients are routinely randomly assigned to the most promising available option(s) or to control arm(s), so that evidence regarding the safest, most effective therapies may be generated in the shortest possible time."[250]

However, the authors also suggest "that although the world was faced with an unknown and frightening disease such as COVID-19 and given concerns over a potentially high case fatality rate, clinicians must maintain a commitment to the rigorous gathering of scientific evidence, in collaboration with global colleagues, so that they may quickly improve outcomes for all patients with COVID-19 worldwide."[251] Where randomized research may not be achievable, specialists must engage in a range of well-designed observational cohort studies as the next best option.

CHAPTER SIX

Recommendations

The pace at which COVID-19 caused significant damage worldwide and especially across the African continent, the USVI, and Haiti, the primary question became: when will this distressing infection end? A vaccine seemed the obvious route to curb increases in cases and stem the tide of transmission. However, even in the wake of vaccine development and distribution, newly discovered variants of the virus and their rapid proliferation suggests COVID-19 could continue spreading until 2022 or further.

According to a report published by the Center for Infectious Disease Research and Policy (CIDRAP), "the pandemic may not end until 60 to 70 percent of the human population becomes immune to the strain and it may take between 18 to 24 months to do so."[252] Mike Osterholm, the report author, and the director of CIDRAP, asserted during an interview with CNN that "the idea that this is going to be done soon defies microbiology."

Researchers applied various models to forecast how COVID-19

will act moving forward, the studies incorporated extensive research and data from previous epidemics before reaching (arriving) at the conclusion.[253] Scientists have compared the COVID-19 outbreak to the 1918 Spanish Flu, which infected 500 million people worldwide. Both viruses are transmitted through droplets emitted when a person coughs or sneezes, passing from one individual - even in the absence of symptoms. The CDC refers to these people as asymptomatic carriers and it estimates that about 40 percent of people infected with coronavirus have mild or no symptoms.[254] In spite of the relatively close similarities, epidemiologists and public health specialists remain reserved on what to expect from COVID-19 moving forward.

One reason for this is the fact that the current strain spreads more easily compared to the 1918 Spanish Flu. An ordinary individual infected with COVID-19 can infect between 2 and 2.5 new people and according to the CIDRAP report there is no way to predict the trajectory of the virus or its variants.[255]

This uncertainty behooves the African continent and Haiti to embrace and prepare for the possibility that a second and bigger trend could be forthcoming.

Recommended Strategies to Avoid Coronavirus Surges:

1 -Continue to keep strict physical social distancing

Social distancing may have to be considered a "new norm" and all social gatherings must be revised. The ideal situation would be that all sports activities, weddings, funerals, birthday gatherings, if possible, must be streamed live and not attended, apart from participants or close family members. However, in rural and remote areas, congested urban areas with ill-developed infrastructure, and areas with poor or no broadband service, this measure may not be feasible, and instead, limitations on the numbers of persons in attendance, coupled with social distancing and the wearing of masks may be the best recourse.

All work locations, colleges, universities, and schools must reconsider how to ensure a safe return, including working and teaching approaches, seating arrangements, toilets and pantries/canteens, and meetings for all the workers and students. To minimize the congestion, schools and universities must plan to designate one-way movement in hallways.

School administrators should discuss having staggered arrival and departure times for students, teachers, and parents so that there would be next to no contact between different groups.

Everywhere, the population must avoid gatherings, reduce physical contact, and practice physical-social distancing at all times outside their homes. Whatever can be done online must be moved there: meetings, shopping, socializing, training, and entertainment. The governments and the population must work together to transform many policies such as rules for elevator usage and achieving social distancing when using escalators.

While necessary, introducing social distancing, at rural and remote areas, even in congested cities, poses unique challenges, as a lack of access to higher quality internet bandwidth for rural residents continues to affect those required to work, conduct school studies from home, and attend other all social gatherings. Specific measures to end the lack of services, combined with infrastructure deficits, including limited access to high-quality bandwidth, might be required to safeguard the quality of life and implement social distancing.

Government and health officials should start by targeting rural and remote areas that may be at higher risk of infection and need resources to fight the pandemic. Rural and remote localities at higher risk could be first in line to receive internet-connected thermometers or more coronavirus tests to provide an early warning of fresh outbreaks.

Broadband can be delivered through fiber, fixed wireless, digital subscriber line (DSL), or cable. A continued lack of resources in those localities will make people less willing to follow public health mandates which could lead to increases in disease cases.

In this strategy, the authorities and the populations at large must reiterate the reality that Jonathan Smith, an infectious disease epidemiologist, enunciates: "people (authorities and populations) should perceive themselves to act as a single individual unit: if one person puts themselves at risk, everyone in the unit is at risk. Once one family member is infected, all are at high risk of infection. Therefore, they have to work as family units to flatten the curve of COVID-19."[256]

2 - Cleaning hands and surfaces must be normative

The message has been loud and clear around the world: washing and sanitizing hands and common surfaces are effective means of thwarting viral transmission. This simple strategy must be encouraged as part of "normal" daily life.

One way to accomplish this is to insist all public places either increase the number of existing sanitizing stations or that such stations be installed. The allocation of government funding to accomplish this will serve as greater encouragement for compliance.

On a personal level, ad campaigns and public service announcements specifying the need to carry and use alcohol-based hand sanitizer must be normative and routine, possibly for years to come.

3 - Wearing masks must become commonplace

At any one time, on any day, a small proportion of the population will have a mild respiratory infection. Therefore, it must become people's norm to wear a mask if they present themselves with a fever, runny nose, or cough, and staying at home if one feels ill should be encouraged and enforced by employers, educators, business owners, etc. and the government.

Employers and teaching organizations must be sensitive to sick people and offer paid leave. Carrying additional masks must be routine and people should think about using them when in a confined space with others who are not close family members, for instance when traveling together. People need to consider all the evidence that is emerging that the routine, widespread use of masks (even proper homemade cloth masks) contributes to reducing the spread of COVID-19 to a considerable extent.

4-Develop rapid-response coronavirus teams ('precision quarantine')

Africa and Haiti will need emergency coronavirus teams that can quickly act when a few cases of an outbreak of COVID-19 or any other virus or highly contagious disease is suspected.

Aggressive contact tracing and the implementation of effective home confinement for people suspected to be sick, must be mandated protocol that is upheld by rapid testing capacity that is enhanced. This type of testing quickly yields results, making people more likely to be tested and treated as results can be provided within one to two hours, if not sooner.

Transfer of those who incur the virus should be conducted as expeditiously as possible to the nearest hospital. Within the health care and treatment setting, the isolation and quarantine of infected patients should be restricted to assigned spaces and areas of the facility with all proper sterile techniques and protocols in place to ensure the virus or disease is contained, minimizing spread so that normal work activities may continue.

It should be recommended that those presenting with mild symptoms remain home and treatment be provided there - including oxygen therapy, if possible.

5-Availability of mass testing capability

The widespread availability of mass rapid testing for identification of symptomatic and asymptomatic persons is a prime necessity as it will help accomplish early quarantine and treatment needs, thereby minimizing spread.

A focus on mass testing for essential workers such as health-care providers, critical clinical workers, teachers, delivery personnel, food service, and grocery store, emergency response personnel, should be decided early. Strategic plans for testing and treatment of all essential staff should be developed with accountability and approval within all government agencies, hospitals, and healthcare facilities and essential businesses. Plans should be submitted to the ministry of public health for review to ensure that outcomes which will benefit all are clearly outlined along with an implementation plan.

6-Use technology to track contacts

The existing interview-based contact tracing is tedious. It would be more effective and efficient to put in place a national hand phone-based contact tracing system similar to those in developed countries such as Singapore.

"Singapore has made its Bluetooth-powered "Trace Together" contact-tracing app its preferred means of recording movements in public spaces across the island. Singapore was one of the first countries to introduce a contact-tracing app, which it had up and running in mid-March 2020. The nation's effort, "Trace Together" used Bluetooth to detect the proximity of other users, recorded such interactions and allowed contact with users in the event they had come into contact with a COVID-carrier. Singapore later added a dedicated Trace Together token that did the same job, but for those who do not or would rather not use a smartphone. In May 2020 Singapore added another system called Safe Entry that required businesses to check visitors into and out of their premises using their smartphones and a QR code."[257, 258]

Granted, individual privacy must be protected, but this must be achieved alongside the need to accelerate contact tracing and inform the population of any exposure and the incumbent need to get tested and/or to self-quarantine for at least two weeks.

Research on best practices for contact tracing that has been successfully conducted in other countries such as Singapore and South Korea, will serve Africa and Haiti well. Application of proven methodologies will ensure contact tracing yields anticipated results and prevent wasting time in developing and testing a system that may not work.

7-All travelers into a country should be screened

More and more nations are re-opening their borders, but some are doing so without requiring screening of travelers entering the country and without sufficient precautions at ports of entry upon arrival. This is a dangerous practice as some of the variants are proving to be more highly transmissible than the initial COVID-19 virus, and there is the strong possibility of a new viral surge occurring.

A COVID-19 PCR test performed at least 3-5 days prior to travel should be required of all travelers and proof of a negative result must be presented upon demand. Airports, docks, and other ports of entry should have established one-way entry and exit, with staff to check test documents. For those who were infected and symptomatic but have recovered, and assuming re-infection does not occur, an antigen test showing antibodies could be formally documented and provided or proof of vaccination cold be required of citizens. However, as has already been stated, as of the writing of this work more than 5,000 cases of COVID-19 have been diagnosed in persons who were fully vaccinated. Hence, proof of vaccination is not proof of not being infected with the virus.

8- All travelers within a country from one city to another should be screened.

While the USVI has made progress containing new sources of infection, the same is not true for Africa and Haiti where new surges are occurring. The continent and Haiti are also experiencing increasing challenges in containing transmission from people traveling within a country from one city to another. Traveling within a country from city to city (especially via shared conveyances such as airplane, bus, or rail) has been shown to increase a person's chance of contracting and spreading COVID-19, including SARS-CoV-2 variants of concern.

Therefore, these areas must take steps necessary to curb the spread of COVID-19, and the following additional recommendations, which could reinforce the existing Travel Advisory issued at the beginning of the outbreaks, could be implemented:

1- If travelers are fully vaccinated:

1-1- Fully vaccinated travelers are less likely to get and spread COVID-19

1-2- People who are fully vaccinated with a WHO- authorized vaccine can travel within a country from city to city and do not need COVID-19 testing or post-travel self-quarantine as long as they continue to take COVID-19 precautions while traveling – wearing a mask, avoiding crowds, socially distancing, and washing hands frequently.

1-3- Fully vaccinated travelers do not need to self-quarantine.

1-4- Fully vaccinated travelers should still follow WHO and country's recommendations for safety.

1-5-1 Wear a mask over their nose and mouth

1-5-2 Stay 6 feet from others or avoid crowds.

1-5-3 Wash their hands often or us hand sanitizer.

2- If travelers are not vaccinated:

If travelers are not fully vaccinated and must travel, they should take the following steps to protect themselves and the others from COVID-19:

2-1 -Before traveling:

2-1-1 Travelers must get tested with a viral test 1-3 days before your trip.

2-2 While they are traveling:

2-2-1 Travelers should wear a mask over their nose and mouth. Masks must be required on planes, buses, trains, and other forms of public transportation traveling into, within, or out of the city and in the country's transportation hubs such as airports and bus or train stations.

2-2-2 Travelers should avoid crowds and stay at least 6 feet away from anyone who is not traveling with them.

2-2-3 Travelers should wash their hands often or use hand sanitizer (with at least 60% alcohol)

2-3 After they travel:

2-3-1 Travelers should get tested with a viral test 3-5 days after travel and self-quarantine for 14 days after travel.

2-3-2 Even if travelers test negative, they should stay home and self-quarantine for 14 days after travel.

2-3-3 If traveler's test is positive, they should isolate themselves to protect others from getting infected.

2-3-4 If travelers did not get tested, they should stay home and self-quarantine for 14 days after travels.

2-3-5 Travelers should avoid being around people who are at increased risk for severe illness for 14 days, whether they get tested or not.

2-3-6 Travelers should self-monitored for COVID-19 symptoms; isolate and get tested if they develop symptoms.

Upon arrival, all travelers should be prepared to undergo enhanced health screening procedures, although several travelers have reported that many countries airports are operating as usual and that even airport employees or flight crew rarely observe social distancing or wear preventative measures such as masks.

3- What to do if you feel unwell

According to the World Health Organization the following must be observed if you feel sick

3-1- Know the full range of symptoms of COVID-19. The most common symptoms of COVID-19 are fever, dry cough, and tiredness. Other symptoms that are less common and may affect some patients include loss of taste or smell, aches and pains, headache, sore throat, nasal congestion, red eyes, diarrhea, or a skin rash.

3-2- Stay home and self-isolate even if you have minor symptoms such as cough, headache, mild fever, until you recover. Call your health care provider or hotline for advice. Have someone bring you supplies. If you need to leave your house or have someone near you, wear a medical mask to avoid infecting others.

3-3- If you have a fever, cough and difficulty breathing, seek medical attention immediately. Call by telephone first if you can and follow the directions of your local health authority.

3-4- Keep up to date on the latest information from trusted sources, such as the WHO or your local and national health authorities. Local and national authorities and public health units are best placed to advise on what people in your area should be doing to protect themselves.

4- Ensure protective and treatment equipment is available in all workplaces where needed.

A significant impediment to fighting the spread of COVID-19 remains the lack of sufficient quantities of personal protective equipment including N-95 and similar respiratory masks, latex and nitrile gloves, hand sanitizer that has a content of at least 60% alcohol, and ventilators.

Funding is the key to assuring PPE and medical equipment is well-supplied. Ample evidence has shown that stockpiles of medical supplies for disasters such as COVID-19 are not adequately funded, leaving storage facilities, particularly hospitals, under-supplied and therefore, ill-equipped to treat patients or to protect staff and providers.

Rather than absolving employers of the accountability to provide this equipment, mandated supply, and enforcement of proper standards for the delivery and continual re-stocking of PPE and medical equipment should be required of employers. Supply chains should be identified, and agreements set in place with alternative plans for delivery in the event primary suppliers are compromised by disaster, illness, shortages, or changes in their own supply chain(s).

Governments should support and provide funding for locally based business entrepreneurs who have the skills to create some PPE such as masks so that facilities are not depending upon a sole source for supplies. Further, identification of multiple suppliers of heavy equipment such as ventilators should be conducted and contracts and agreements for emergency service and supply should be pre-arranged so that there is no delay when needed.

5- Provide workers' compensation for employees who contract COVID-19 on the job

Evidence shows that employee compensation programs administered by many African nations, Haiti, and the USVI during this COVID-19 crisis suffered substantial decreases or losses in the few benefits they offered. This resulted in thousands of employees who had contracted COVID-19 in the course of performing their job duties, falling into poverty due to the loss of wages and high hospital and medical bills.

According to the UN Human Rights Council report "More than 70 million people are expected to fall into extreme poverty because of COVID-19."[259] Another published report from the United Nations Economic Commission for Africa (UNECA) projected "that the ongoing COVID-19 pandemic could push 29 million people into extreme poverty across Africa."[260]

It is unfortunate that instead of strategizing true economic recovery and support for workers, many African governments and the government of Haiti have placed more emphasis on presenting the appearance of resuming economic normalcy. This pretense incorrectly conflates lifting partial or total restriction directives with the measures that would be required to give the populations the confidence to resume activity fully and safely and benefit real economic recovery.

Many African nations centered their compensation for economic legislation on policies that forced employees to accept risky working conditions to preserve their incomes. This approach follows on the failure, to date, not only to put in place measures to protect the essential workers who have been working on the front lines throughout this pandemic, but also to compensate those who cannot prove having contracted COVID-19 during their work. The message sent by this stance by government and employers is that the lives of employees are insignificant. This attitude does not engender trust when people are told or asked to comply with mandates they believe have been constructed by government and employers to whom their health and safety are unimportant.

There are some nations in Africa and around the world that have made it easier for essential workers and/or health care workers to gain employee compensation by establishing policies or procedures wherein contracting COVID-19 in the workplace is a presumed probability due to the nature of work being performed or the work environment. Unfortunately, this is not a practice undertaken by every African nation or Haiti. A key recommendation to ameliorate this problem is that governments should consider passing legislation establishing a compensation program to pay benefits to employees who contract COVID-19 at work in full or at least up to two-thirds of their regular pay. Such legislation would not just support those employees at the greatest threat of contracting the virus or who already contracted the virus at work, it would also protect the wider communities from the spread of COVID-19 as these employees could then afford to remain at home or seek treatment, and such compensation would put the economies on a brighter foundation for everybody.

6-Other approaches needed to return to a normal life.

Improving public health services that have been abandoned for decades, enhancing medical facilities to increase intensive care bed capacity, providing economic support, and stimulus for the population, employing proven strategies to address recession and job loss, improving, and expanding safety nets and social supports to all the population, especially for the vulnerable - these measures would enhance the viability and recovery of COVID-19 stricken nations.

The Delta Variant of COVID-19: New Concerns

Herd immunity to a pathogen is reached when a specified percentage of a population is immune to that pathogen and they and the remainder of the populous can then avoid sustained transmission. The threshold is regulated by several factors, including the transmissibility of the illness.[261] More infectious strains of SARS-CoV-2 raise the expectation on herd immunity as the virus has been mutating since being discovered a year ago.

The troubling development in recent months has been the confirmation of a new COVID-19 variant strain known as Delta. Initially identified as B.1.617.2, the Delta variant is the most contagious version of the COVID-19 virus to date. First detected in India, in December 2020, where it rapidly exhausted that country's health care system, it has now been recorded in 124 countries including Africa, the USVI, and Haiti. The variant strain already accounts for over three-quarters of sequenced specimens in many major countries, according to the WHO and other published reports."[262-264]

Although effective data are still emerging, preliminary evaluations show that the transmissibility rate of the Delta variant is higher than that of the earlier SARS-CoV-2 strain and may also be higher among children as well.[265, 266] The WHO asserts that "the highly contagious Delta variant of COVID-19 is expected to become the dominant strain of the virus over the coming months."[267] The UN health agency, in its weekly epidemiological report, corroborated this assertion by stating that "the Delta variant of COVID-19 is expected to out-compete, rapidly, other variants and become the dominant circulating lineage over the coming months."[268]

The International Health Organization believes that "overall, 3.4 million new COVID-19 cases were reported in July 18 – up 12% from the week before and at this rate the cumulative number of cases reported globally could exceed 200 million in the next three weeks." "And that the global increases in transmission appeared to be driven by four factors: more transmissible variants; the relaxation of public health measures; increased social mixing and large numbers of unvaccinated people."[269]

As of today, there is not yet any sign of a higher rate of mortality with the Delta variant strain. However, there are concerns that the new strain could affect how antibodies combine to the disease and could decrease the effectiveness of vaccines or antibody treatments developed over the past few months.

According to the WHO "the COVID-19 vaccines that are currently in development or have been approved, are expected to provide at least some protection against new virus_variants because these vaccines elicit a broad immune response involving a range of antibodies and cells. Therefore, changes or mutations in the virus should not make vaccines completely ineffective. In the event that any of these vaccines prove to be less effective against one or more variants, it will be possible to change the composition of the vaccines to protect against these variants."[270]

The Delta variant is expected to continue propagating in the coming months, driven by its reproductive advantage over the original COVID-19 variant SARS-CoV-2.

There is substantial new data evidencing that the Pfizer-BioN-Tech, Moderna, and Johnson & Johnson vaccines for COVID-19 are successful at protecting against the Delta variant strain. Therefore, it is vitally important that Africa, USVI, and Haitian governments and public health authorities encourage people to get vaccinated and continue to take precautions, such as masking and social distancing.

However, it does not help that nations such as Haiti, offered the vaccine via the WHO's COVAX program, did not have preparations in place to receive the vaccines as late as June 2021, leaving the environment open to continued proliferation of the virus and any variants.[271-272] The island nation finally accepted COVAX vaccines from the United States on July 14, 2021[273]

If the world, not just individual nations, is to combat and win against this virus, then every nation must obtain vaccines and launch aggressive campaigns to get as many people as possible vaccinated in order that the globe may experience herd immunity at last. Many countries are reopening businesses and resuming operations because of the fear that economies will suffer; but the truth is if sufficient numbers of people are not vaccinated, there is every possibility that economies will suffer even more due to the loss of life and the extended time people will have to take off due to illness.

This is a global issue that demands the attention, fortitude, and the united approach of all nations. Viruses mutate. With each mutation, a new and tougher variant can arise. Consequently, the best approach to avoid the possible negative and detrimental effects of a new variant mutation is to vaccinate as many people as possible to achieve herd immunity.

According to the WHO report, *Vaccines Explained*, vaccines are a critical tool in the battle against COVID-19, and there are clear public health and lifesaving benefits to using the tools we already have. We must not put off getting vaccinated because of our concerns about new variants, and we must proceed with vaccination even if the vaccines may be somewhat less effective against some of the COVID-19 virus variants. We need to use the tools we have in hand even while we continue to improve those tools. We are all safe only if everyone is safe.[274]

Determinants That Could Minimize COVID-19 Related Deaths

1 - Immunity through COVID-19 vaccine

Rolling out an efficient COVID-19 and Delta variant vaccine in high-risk populations could considerably decrease related deaths.

2 - Cross- immunity

Possible T-cell cross-reactivity immunity of SARS-CoV-2 and other coronaviruses being examined. Understanding how pre-existing specific T cells that are present in the general population affect the susceptibility to and pathogenesis of SARS-CoV-2 infection is important for the management of the current COVID-19 pandemic.

3 - Immunity through other vaccines

Potential correlation between Bacille Calmette-Guerin (BCG) vaccination and the reduction of COVID-19 and Delta variant case counts and related mortality being examined.

According to an article published in the US. National Library of Medicine National Institute of Health, which has analyzed the SARS-CoV-2 genomes "Bacillus Calmette–Guérin vaccine, can elicit trained innate immunity and confer protection against COVID-19."[275-276]

The evidence continues to suggest that gained immunity through other vaccines presents considerable protection against the new variants now spreading worldwide.

The expectation is that gained immunity from the vaccines will certainly deliver long-lasting protection against SARS-CoV-2 and bring an end to the deadly disease.

4 - The decreased rate of transmission

Rapid detection of COVID-19 and its Delta variant through fast and accurate testing, followed by immediate quarantine actions, could decrease associated deaths, and allow faster resumption of activities

5 - Better treatment

Enhanced understanding of COVID-19 and the Delta variant and improvements in treatments could reduce related deaths. Assessing and identifying effective vaccine candidates for human use is crucial for prioritizing vaccination programs against COVID-19. The sequential immunization strategy that has been studied for many infectious disease vaccines might help mitigate many of the shortcomings of the current lot of COVID-19 vaccines. Further research should be conducted to investigate the impact of these variants on vaccination, and new vaccines targeting the important new variants (such as 501Y. V2), should at least be researched, prepared, and made available immediately.

6 - Natural Immunity

A more considerable population with COVID-19 immunity through exposure could lower associated deaths. The fundamental concept behind this approach is to let low-risk people socialize and naturally become infected with the coronavirus, while vulnerable people would maintain social distancing and continue to shelter in place. Therefore, "natural herd immunity" will develop and reduce harm from SARS-CoV-2 while protecting everyone. Once this process occurs, infected individuals can no longer spread the disease, and the epidemic will burn out.

Another route to get herd immunity should be through mass vaccination, as developed countries, including many African nations have done with measles, smallpox, and largely with polio.

Although there is growing optimism and hope with this approach, achieving herd immunity against COVID-19 could be also challenging as there is much skepticism about the prospect and occurrence of the emergence of new variants, the reduction in vaccine efficacy for each variant, the critical question of cross-variant immunity, and the consistency of safe human behavior. Until then, mass SARS-CoV-2 vaccination, social distancing, and use of face coverings, with comprehensive case identification, testing, tracing, and isolation, are the safest approach.

Conclusion

I wrote this book intending to start a conversation about the negative impact the delusional denials and distortion of the COVID-19 deadly virus had on populations and countries at large. The COVID-19 outbreak will not be stopped for one fraction of a second by delusional denials, distortion, or ruse; instead, it will only be defeated by strictly unbiased measures that prevent its spread, while at the same time allowing people to live productive lives.

China and some other more developed countries have been able to slow the spread of COVID-19 by acting objectively and enforcing proven effective measures such as lockdowns of homes and enforced closures of city and regional borders (known as cordon sanitaire). These measures although stringent, are highly effective.

Deplorably, the African continent and Haiti are now undergoing a worsening increase of confirmed cases and deaths because most of their population and some of their leading figures continue to engage in distortion and denial even as a more highly transmissible and contagious variant makes its way across their paths. If recommendations for improved identification of cases and treatment, funding for PPE and medical equipment, and succinct and targeted messaging and education about the virus, and preventive mandates for public interaction are not put in place, enforced, and modeled by those in authority, not only will denial, distortion and delusion continue, but the number of cases and deaths will continue to rise.

The hard-core reality is that even if COVID-19 eventually goes dormant or the world's populations reach protective herd immunity levels, there will be another pandemic, another epidemic that rages out of control, crosses borders, is spread by travelers and becomes a pandemic. Epidemics and pandemics are part of our world. Travel and the transport and domestication of animals keep disease and vermin spreading throughout the world. This means the only viable and pragmatic solutions are to

1. Learn from past incidents.
2. Cull best practices from other countries and adapt and adopt them.
3. Share knowledge, techniques, methodologies, and strategies.
4. Increase and guarantee funding (with accountability measures and enforcement processes) for PPE and medical equipment.
5. Design and implement compensation programs and packages for employees and the self-employed.
6. Put together planning teams consisting of stakeholders

from government, private enterprise, local community, representatives for the elderly and the developmentally and physically challenged.

7. With planning teams, create plans for preparedness, response, and recovery from pandemics, catastrophic public health events.
8. Work with countries known for excellent emergency management to develop procedures and processes to exercise plans on a regular basis.
9. Commit to improving existing health care systems and infrastructure
10. Establish accountability measures to ensure data is gathered, reported, and corroborated honestly both within the country and with other nations. Africa and Haiti must put aside false pride in reporting data that makes them look good. Such reporting is to the detriment of their people as inaccurate reporting stymies any aide for which they may qualify from international sources.

If governments in African nations, Haiti, and the USVI will seriously employ the suggestions made herein along with others that are equally viable, the problems with delusional myths and denial of disease existence and transmission, will be controlled and have less of an effect on population compliance with public health prevention measures. More importantly, they will be better prepared to respond to and effectively survive the next pandemic.

References For COVID-19 Book

[1] WHO Coronavirus Disease (COVID-19) Dashboard; retrieved from https://covid19.who.int.

[2] Almeida, J.D., Berry, D.M., Cunningham, C.H., Hamre, D., Hofstad, M.S., Mallucci, L., McIntosh, K. and Tyrrell, D.A. (1968) Virology: Coronaviruses. Nature, 220, 650. https://doi.org/10.1038/220650b0

[3] Column: The lab-leak origin claim for COVID-19 is in the news, but it is still fact-free; retrieved from www.latimes.com/business/story/2021-06-03/lab-leak-covid-origin

[4] Coronavirus: Is there any evidence for lab release theory? Retrieved from www.bbc.com/news/science-environment-52318539

[5] The Lab-Leak Hypothesis. Retrieved from www.

nymag.com/intelligencer/article/coronavirus-lab-escape-theory.html

[6] SARS. WHO, Emergencies preparedness, response. Retrieved from https://www.who.int/csr/sars/country/2003_07_11/en/

[7] Global research on coronavirus disease (COVID-19). Retrieved from https://www.who.int/emergencies/diseases/novel-coronavirus-2019/global-research-on-novel-coronavirus-2019-ncov

[8] Corona Virus: A General Introduction. Centre for Evidence Based Medicine, Nuffield Department of Primary Care Health Sciences University of Oxford: https://www.cebm.net/covid-19/coronaviruses-a-general-introduction.

[9] Animals are still key to preventing the next pandemic; retrieved from https://www.axios.com/animals-prevent-pandemic-task-force-25151abd-f274-4931-a1d5-a44a9d2428fa.html

[10] Intelligence Community Statement on Origins of COVID-19. Press Release (2020);

retrieved from https://www.dni.gov/index.php/newsroom/press-releases/item/2112-intelligence-community-statement-on-origins-of-covid-19?tmpl=component&print=1

[11] Column: The lab-leak origin claim for COVID-19 is in the news, but it is still fact-free https://www.latimes.com/business/story/2021-06-03/lab-leak-covid-origin /

[12] Coronavirus: Is there any evidence for lab release theory? https://www.bbc.com/news/science-environment-52318539

[13] The Lab-Leak Hypothesis. https:// www. nymag.com/intelligencer/article/coronavirus-lab-escape-theory.html

[14] de Groot R.J., Baker S.C., Baric R.S. Middle East Respiratory Syndrome Coronavirus (MERS-Cov); Announcement of the Coronavirus Study Group. J Virol. Virol. 2013 Jul; 87(14): 7790–7792. doi: 10.1128/JVI.01244-13 https://www.ncbi.nlm.nih.gov/pmc/articles/PMC3700179/pdf/zjv7790.pdf/?tool=EBI

[15] Zaki, A.M., van Boheemen S., Bestebroer T.M.,

Osterhaus A.D., Fouchier R.A. Isolation of a novel coronavirus from a man with pneumonia in Saudi Arabia. N Engl J Med. 2012; 367:1814-1820 DOI: 10.1056/NEJMoa1211721 https:// www.nejm.org/doi/10.1056/NEJMoa1211721?url_ver=Z39.88-2003&rfr_id=ori%3Arid%3Acrossref.org&rfr_dat=cr_pub++0www.ncbi.nlm.nih.gov

[16] Fineberg H.V. Pandemic preparedness and response-lessons from H1N1influenza of 2009.N Engl J Med.2014; 370:1335-1342 DOI: 10.1056/NEJMra1208802 https:// www.nejm.org/doi/10.1056/NEJMra1208802?url_ver=Z39.88-2003&rfr_id=ori:rid:crossref.org&rfr_dat=cr_pub%20%200www.ncbi.nlm.nih.gov

[17] Hayden F.G. Respiratory viral threats. Curr Opin Dis. 2006.
How COVID-19 is Spread. Published online 2013 Feb 22. doi: 10.1186/1471-2334-13-97
https://www.ncbi.nlm.nih.gov/pmc/articles/PMC3606325/
https://www.bmcinfectdis.biomedcentral.com/track/pdf/10.1186/1471-2334-13-97.pdf

[18] Severe acute respiratory syndrome (SARS). https://

www.cdc.gov/sars/about/faq.html.

[19] World Health Organization. Annex C: Respiratory droplets. In: Atkinson J., Chartier Y., Pessoa-Silva C.L., editors. Natural ventilation for infection control in health-care settings. WHO; Geneva: 2009. Retrieved from https://www.ncbi.nlm.nih.gov/books/NBK143284/ https:// www.pubmed.ncbi.nlm.nih.gov/23762969/

[20] Bridges C.B., Kuehnert M.J., Hall C.B. Transmission of influenza: implications for control in health care settings. Clin Infect Dis. 2003. Retrieved from https:// pubmed.ncbi.nlm.nih.gov/14523774/

[21] Boone S.A., Gerba C.P. Significance of fomites in the spread of respiratory and enteric viral disease. Appl Environ Microbiol. 2007. Published online 2007 Jan 12. doi: 10.1128/AEM.02051-06/ https://www.ncbi.nlm.nih.gov/pmc/articles/PMC1828811/

[22] Brankston G., Gitterman L., Hirji Z., Lemieux C., Gardam M. Transmission of influenza A in human beings. Lancet Infect Dis.2007. Apr;7(4):257-65. doi: 10.1016/S1473-3099(07)70029-4. https:// www.pubmed.ncbi.nlm.nih.gov/17376383/ https:// www.thelancet.com/journals/laninf/article/PIIS1473-3099(07)70029-4/fulltext

[23] Bean B., Moore B.M., Sterner B., Petersen L.R., Gerding D.N., Balfour H.H., Jr. Survival of influenza viruses on environmental surfaces. J Infect Dis. Dis1982 Jul;146(1):47-51.doi: 10.1093/infdis/146.1.47./ https:// www.pubmed.ncbi.nlm.nih.gov/6282993/
Also recorded in, *The Journal of Infectious Diseases*, Volume 146, Issue 1, July 1982, Pages 47 51, https://doi.org/10.1093/infdis/146.1.47 https://www.academic.oup.com/jid/articleabstract/ 146/1/47/992812?redirectedFrom=fulltext

[24] Otter, J. A., Donskey, C., Yezli, S., Douthwaite, S., Goldenberg, S. D., & Weber, D. J. (2016). Transmission of SARS and MERS coronaviruses and influenza virus in healthcare settings: the possible role of dry surface contamination. The Journal of hospital infection, 92(3), 235–250. https://doi.org/10.1016/j.jhin.2015.08.027

[25] vanDoremalenN., BushmaketT., MunsterV,J.Stability of Middle East respiratory syndrome coronavirus (MERS-CoV) under different environmental conditions; PMID: 24084338 DOI: 10.2807/1560-7917.es2013.18.38.20590 https:// www.pubmed.ncbi.nlm.nih.gov/24084338/ https://www.eurosurveillance.org/ content/10.2807/1560-7917.ES2013.18.38.20590 https:// www.eurosurveillance.org/images/dynamic/

EE/V18N38/art20590.pdf

[26] Chan K.H., Peiris J.S., Lam S.Y., Poon L.L., K.Y., Seto W.H. The effects of temperature and relative humidity on the viability of the SARS Coronavirus. Adv Virol. 2011. Published online 2011 Oct 1. doi: 10.1155/2011/734690 https://www.ncbi.nlm.nih.gov/pmc/articles/PMC3265313/

[27] Coulliette A.D., Perry K.A., Edwards J.R., Noble-Wang J.A. Persistence of the 2009 pandemic influenza A(H1N1) virus on N95 respirators. Appl Environ Microbiol. 2013. PMID: 23335770 PMCID: PMC3623216 DOI: 10.1128/AEM.03850-12
https://www.ncbi.nlm.nih.gov/pmc/articles/PMC3623216/

[28] Boone S. A., Gerba C.P. Significance of fomites in the spread of respiratory and enteric viral disease. Apple Environ Microbiol. 2007. Published online 2007 Jan 12. doi: 10.1128/AEM.02051-06 https:// www.ncbi.nlm.nih.gov/pmc/articles/PMC1828811/
https://www.journals.asm.org/doi/full/10.1128/AEM.02051-06

[29] Musher D.M. How contagious are common respiratory

tract infections? N Engl J Med. 2003; 348:1256-1266 DOI: 10.1056/NEJMra02177 https://www.nejm.org/doi/10.1056/NEJMra021771?url_ver=Z39.88-2003&rfr_id=ori:rid:crossref.org&rfr_dat=cr_pub%20%200pubmed

[30] Gwaltney J.M., Jr., Hendley J.O. Transmission of experimental rhinovirus by contaminated surfaces. Am J Epidemiol. 1982. American Journal of Epidemiology, Volume 116, Issue 5, November 1982, Pages 828 833, doi.org/10.1093/oxfordjournals.aje.a113473 https://www.academic.oup.com/aje/articleabstract/116/5/828/111471?redirectedFrom=fulltext

[31] Abad F.X., Pinto R.M., Borsch A. Survival of enteric viruses on environmental fomites. Appl Environ Microbiol. 1994; Oct;60(10):3704-10. ·doi: 10.1128/aem.60.10.3704-3710.1994.https:// www.ncbi.nlm.nih.gov/pmc/articles/PMC201876/pdf/aem00027-0234.pdf https:// www.ncbi.nlm.nih.gov/pmc/articles/PMC201876/

[32] Hall C.B. Respiratory syncytial virus: its transmission in the hospital environment. Yale J Biol Med. 1982; May-Aug 1982;55(3-4):219-23. https:// www.ncbi.nlm.nih.

gov/pmc/articles/PMC2596445/
https:// www. pubmed.ncbi.nlm.nih.gov/6758370/

[33] CDC expands definition of who is a 'close contact' of an individual with covid-19
https://www.washingtonpost.com/health/2020/10/21/coronavirus-close-contact-cdc/
https://www.cdc.gov/coronavirus/2019-ncov/php/contact-tracing/contact-tracing-plan/appendix.html#contact
https://www.cdc.gov/coronavirus/2019-ncov/php/contact-tracing/contact-tracing-plan/contact-tracing.html

[34] 75% emerging infectious diseases zoonotic: UN Report. https://www.downtoearth.org.in/news/health/75-emerging-infectious-diseases-zoonotic-un-report-72173

[35] Prioritizing and preventing deadly zoonitc diseases. Retrieved from https://www.cdc.gov/globalhealth/healthprotection/fieldupdates/winter-2017/prevent-zoonotic-diseases.html

[36] Zoonotic diseases (also known as zoonoses) are caused by germs that spread between animals and people. https://www.cdc.gov/onehealth/basics/zoonotic-diseases.html / 8 Zoonotic Diseases Shared

[37] Between Animals and People of Most Concern in the U.S. https://www.cdc.gov/media/releases/2019/s0506-zoonotic-diseases-shared.html

[38] What you should know aboutCOVID-19 and pets. Retrieved from https://www.cdc.gov/coronavirus/2019-ncov/daily-life-coping/pets.html

[39] https://www.worldometers.info/coronavirus/worldwide-graphs/#total-deaths

[40] Hamill, Jasper. (2020). Coronavirus has an 'HIV-like mutation' which helps it attack human cells, scientists claim.Retrievedfromhttps://metro.co.uk/2020/02/27/coronavirus-hiv-like-mutation-helps-attack-human-cells-scientists-claim-12314129/?ito=cbshare

[41] Coronavirus could attack immune system like HIV by targeting protective cells, warn scientists. Retrieved from https://www.scmp.com/news/china/society/article/3079443/coronavirus-could-target-immune-system-targeting-protective

[42] (2020). Coronavirus could attack immune system like HIV by targeting protective cells, warn scientists.

Retrieved from https://www.todayonline.com/world/coronavirus-could-attack-immune-system-hiv-targeting-protective-cells-warn-scientists

[43] (2021). China claims to have found 24 different previously – unknown coronaviruses in bats as it fights back against growing lab leak suspicions. Retrieved from https://www.dailymail.co.uk/news/article-9676127/China-claims-24-different-new-coronaviruses-bats-amid-lab-leak-suspicions.html

[44] Karlis, Nicole. (2020). Why COVID-19 is more insidious than other coronaviruses. Retrieved from https://www.salon.com/2020/02/27/why-covid-19-is-more-insidious-than-other-coronaviruses/

[45] Why COVID-19 is more insidious than other coronaviruses. The "genomic packing" mechanism of COVID-19 may be more like Ebola and HIV, researchers in the US and China say
https://www.scmp.com/news/china/society/article/3052495/coronavirus-far-more-likely-sars-bond-human-cells-scientists-say

[46] IBID

[47] The CoronaVac's genetic code is 80 percent similar to SARS. https:// www. thehill.com/changing-america/well-being/ prevention-cures/481455-the-coronaviruss- genetic-code-is-80-percent SARS-CoV-2

[48] An Update on Genomics, Risk Assessment, Potential Therapeutics and Vaccine Development. https:// www. ncbi.nlm.nih.gov/pmc/articles/PMC7915969/

[49] Structure of Furin Protease Binding to SARS-CoV-2 Spike Glycoprotein and Implications for Potential Targets and Virulence. https:/www.ncbi.nlm.nih.gov/ pmc/articles/PMC7409919/

[50] Park, J. E. et al. Proteolytic processing of Middle East respiratory syndrome coronavirus spikes expands virus tropism. Proc. Natl Acad. Sci. USA 113, 12262–12267 (2016). https:// www.nature.com/articles/s41564-021-00908-w

[51] Johnson, B. A. et al. Loss of furin cleavage site attenuates SARS-CoV-2 pathogenesis. Nature https://doi. org/10.1038/s41586-021-03237-4 (2021). https:// www. nature.com/articles/s41564-021-00908-w

[52] Romeu, A.R.; Ollé, E. SARS-CoV-2 and the Secret of the Furin Site. Preprints 2021, 2021020264 (doi: 10.20944/preprints202102.0264.v1). Retrieved from https://www.preprints.org/manuscript/202102.0264/v1

[53] The origin of the SARS-CoV-2 furin cleavage site remains a mystery. Retrieved from https://www.news-medical.net/news/20210217/The-origin-of-SARS-CoV-2-furin-cleavage-site-remains-a-mystery.aspx

[54] Hallenberger S, Bosch V, Angliker H, Shaw E, Klenk HD, Garten W (Nov 1992). "Inhibition of furin-mediated cleavage activation of HIV-1 glycoprotein gp160". Nature, htpps:// www.pubmed.ncbi.nlm.nih.gov/1360148/

[55] Furin cleavage site in the SARS-CoV-2 coronavirus glycoprotein. https:// www.virology.ws/2020/02/13/furin-cleavage-site-in-the-sars-cov-2-coronavirus-glycoprotein/

[56] Furin cleavage site in the SARS-CoV-2 coronavirus glycoprotein.
https://www.virology.ws/2020/02/13/furin-cleavage-site-in-the-sars-cov-2-coronavirus-glycoprotein/

[57] COVID-19, SARS, and MERS: are they closely related? Published online 2020 Mar 28. doi: 10.1016/j.cmi.2020.03.026 https://www.ncbi.nlm.nih.gov/pmc/articles/PMC7176926/

[58] Center for Disease Control and Prevention (CDC) website:https://www.cdc.gov/coronavirus/2019-ncov/symptoms-testing/symptoms.html#self-checker.

[59] The First, Second, And Third World Countries: Origin Of Concept And Present Beliefs https://www.worldatlas.com/articles/the-first-second-and-third-world-countries-origin-of-concept-and-present-beliefs.html

[60] Why are countries classified as First, Second or Third World? https://www.history.com/news/why-are-countries-classified-as-first-second-or-third-world

[61] Countries of the Third World. https://www.nationsonline.org/oneworld/third_world.htm

[62] Is the term 'developing world' outdated? https://www.weforum.org/agenda/2015/11/is-the-term-developing-world-outdated/

[63] COVID-19 in Africa: the spread and response. https:// www.nature.com/articles/s41591-020-0961-x/

[64] China moves to smooth relations with African students. https://www.timeshighereducation.com/news/china-moves-smooth-relations-african-students.

[65] Why Africa loves China. https:// www.aljazeera.com/opinions/2019/1/6/why-africa-loves-china/.

[66] There are more African students than ever in China. Why are they still alienated? https:// www.studyinternational.com/news/african-students-china-alienated/

[67] Gilbert M. et al. Lancet (2020), Preparedness and vulnerability of African countries against importations of COVID-19: a modelling study. htpps:// www.thelancet.com/pdfs/journals/lancet/PIIS0140-6736(20)30411-6.pdf.

[68] Preparedness and vulnerability of African countries against importations of COVID-19: a modelling study. htpps:// www.pubmed.ncbi.nlm.nih.gov/32087820/

[69] Menkir, T.F., Chin, T., Hay, J.A. et al. Estimating

internationally imported cases during the early COVID-19 pandemic. Nat Commun 12, 311 (2021). doi.org/10.1038/s41467-020-20219-8

[70] Estimating internationally imported cases during the early COVID-19 pandemic. htpps:// www.nature.com/articles/s41467-020-20219-8

[71] Africa: Covid-19 - How Five Hardest Hit African Countries are Coping; retrieved from https://allafrica.com/stories/202102210058.html

[72] COVID-19:Situation update for the WHO African Region 27 May 2020; retrieved from https://apps.who.int/iris/bitstream/handle/10665/332199/SITREP_COVID-19_WHOAFRO_20200527-eng.pdf

[73] Countries with the most COVID-19 (Coronavirus) cases; retrieved from Countries With the Most COVID-19 (Coronavirus) Cases - TheTopTens

[74] Marguerite Massinga Loembé, Akhona Tshangela, Stephanie J. Salyer, Jay K. Varma, Ahmed E. Ogwell Ouma & John N. Nkengasong COVID-19 in Africa: the spread and response. https:// www.nature.com/articles/s41591-020-0961-x/

[75] COVID-19:Situation update for the WHO African Region 27 May 2020; retrieved from https://apps.who.int/iris/bitstream/handle/10665/332199/SITREP_COVID-19_WHOAFRO_20200527-eng.pdf

[76] WHO Coronavirus Disease (COVID-19) Dashboard. Retrieved f from:
https://covid19.who.int.

[77] Why is COVID-19 more deadly than Ebola? An infectious disease doctor explains. Retrieved from https://www.forbes.com/sites/coronavirusfrontlines/2020/07/31/why-is-covid-19-more-deadly-than-ebola-an-infectious-disease-doctor-explains/?sh=2b3282f4f734

[78] The Corona Virus Disease 2019 (Covid-19) Strategic Response Plan For the WHO African Region. https://www.afro.who.int/sites/default/files/2020-06/SPRP%20BUDGET%200520_01.pdf

[79] Coronavirus: How Fast Is It Spreading In Africa retrieved from
https://www.peacefmonline.com/pages/local/health/202007/418048.php

[80] Coronavirus: How fast is it spreading in Africa? retrieved from https://www.ghanaweb.com/GhanaHomePage/africa/Coronavirus-How-fast-is-it-spreadi Africa-1001263

[81] Massinga Loembé, M., Tshangela, A., Salyer, S.J. et al. COVID-19 in Africa: the spread and response. Nat Med 26, 999–1003 (2020); retrieved from https://doi.org/10.1038/s41591-020-0961-x

[82] Centers for Disease Control and Prevention (CDC): retrieved from https://www.cdc.gov/foodsafety/outbreaks/investigating-outbreaks/epi-curves.html

[83] Naicker S, Plange-Rhule J, Tutt RC, Eastwood JB. Shortage of healthcare workers in developing countries--Africa. Ethn Dis. 2009 Spring;19(1 Suppl 1):S1-60-4. PMID: 19484878.

[84] Ighobor, Kinsley; (2017) Diagnosing Africa's medical brain drain: Higher wages and modern facilities are magnets for Africa's health workers. Retrieved from https://www.un.org/africarenewal/magazine/december-2016-march-2017/diagnosing-africa%E2%80%99s-medical-brain-drain

[85] Africa's changing demographics https://www.brookings.edu/blog/brookings-now/2019/01/18/charts-of-the-week-africas-changing-demographics.

[86] Foresight Africa: Top proprieties for the continent in 2019. Retrieved from https://www.brookings.edu/multi-chapter-report/foresight-africa-top-priorities-for-the-continent-in-2019.

[87] More young people infected with Covid-19 as cases surge globally | World news | The Guardian. Retrieved from https://www.theguardian.com/world/2020/jun/26/more-young-people-infected-with-covid-19-as-cases-surge-globally

[88] https://2020census.gov/en/conducting-the-count/island-areas/virgin-islands.html.

[89] Virgin Islands Struggle while Puerto Rico Rebounds. Retrieved from https://libertystreeteconomics.newyorkfed.org/2019/10/us-virgin-islands-struggle-while-puerto-rico-rebounds.html

[90] Retrieved from https://www.bloomberg.com/news/articles/2019-10-02/hurricane-recovery-in-u-s-virgin-islands-lags-puerto-rico-s

[90] U. S. Virgin Islands Economy 2020. Retrieved from https://theodora.com/wfbcurrent/virgin_islands/virgin_islands_economy.html

[91] Health Care in Puerto Rico and the U.S. Virgin Islands: A Six-Month Check-Up After the Storms (Report). Retrieved from https:// www.kff.org/medicaid/issue-brief/health-care-in-puerto-rico-and-the-u-s-virgin-islands-a-six-month-check-up-after-the-storms-report/

[92] Muhammad Abdul Baker Chowdhury et al. 2019. Health Impact of Hurricanes Irma and Maria on St Thomas and St John, US Virgin Islands, 2017–2018. https://www.ajph.aphapublications.org/doi/full/10.2105/AJPH.2019.305310

[93] IntheU.S.VirginIslands,HealthCareRemainsInACritical State. https://www.npr.org/2018/02/04/582256476/in-the-u-s-virgin-islands-health-care-remains-in-a-critical-state

[94] Governor Bryan to Updates Residents on COVID-19. Retrieved from https://www.vi.gov/governor-bryan-updates-residents-on-covid-19-3/

[95] https://www.covid19usvi.com/what-us-virgin-

islands-department-health-doing-about-COVID-19.

[96] USVI COVID-19 Timeline; retrieved from https://www.vi.gov/usvi-covid-19-timeline/

[97] https://www.vi.gov/covid

[98] WHO Coronavirus Disease (COVID-19) Dashboard. https://covid19.who.int

[99] People with Certain Medical Conditions. https://. www.cdc.gov/coronavirus/2019-ncov/need-extra-precautions/people-with-medicalconditions.html?CDC.

[100] Increased Risk of Severe Illness from COVID-19 https:// www.cdc.gov/coronavirus/2019-ncov/need-extra-precautions/older-adults.html.

[101] Sarah LaFave (2020). The impact of COVID-19 on older adults.
https://www.hub.jhu.edu/2020/05/05/impact-of-covid-19-on-the-elderly/

[102] St. Croix History and General Information. https://www.stcroixtourism.com/aboutstcroix.htm

[103] St. Croix: Facts & History. Retrieved from https:// www.vinow.com/ stcroix/ history

[104] About St. Croix. https:/ / www.visitstcroix.com/ island-overview.html

[105] Limetree Bay Activates COVID-19 Response Plan After Confirmation of First Related Case in Village. Retrieved from https: / / www.doh.vi.gov / NewsRelease_032320_ Limetree20COVID-19 2019Positive.pdf

[106] Limetree Bay Activates COVID-19 Response Plan After Confirmation of First Related Case in Village. Retrieved from https:/ / www.doh.vi.gov / news/ limetree-bay-activates-covid-19-response-plan-after-confirmation-first-related-case-village.

[107] O'Hare, Marueen & Hardingham-Gil, / /tamara (2020). Coronavirus: Which countries have travel bans? Retrieved from https:/ / edition.cnn.com/ travel/ article/ coronavirus-travel-bans/ index.html

[108] MacDonald, Isabel (2020). "Irresponsible and Dangerous": U.S. deports Haitians despite coronavirus

risks. Retrieved from https://theintercept.com/2020/04/12/haiti-coronavirus-united-states-deportation

[109] Reuters staff (2020). Haiti declares emergency over coronavirus, imposes curfew, shuts borders. Retrieved from https://reuters.com/article/us-health-coronavirus-haiti-idUSKBN21700V

[110] Paultre, Andre & Marsh, Sarah (2020). Haiti to reopen textile factories despite coronavirus fears. Retrieved from: https://www.usnews.com/news/world/articles/2020-04-15/haiti-to-reopen-textile-factories-despite-coronavirus-fears

[111] Medecins Sans Frontieres/Doctors Without Borders (2020). Haiti: MSF raises alarm over rapid spike in new cases of COVID-19. Retrieved from https://www.doctorswithoutborders.org/what-we-do/news-stories/news/haiti-msf-raises-alarm-over-rapid-spike-new-cases-covid-19

[112] COVID-19: Only PCR Tests Are Authorized For Screening in Haiti. Retrieved from https://haitiantimes.com/2020/06/18/covid-19-only-pcr-tests-are-authorized-for-screeningin-haiti/

[113] Overall total population" – World Population Prospects: The 2019 Revision" (xslx). population.un.org (custom data gained via the website). United Nations Department of Economic and Social Affairs, Population Division 2019. (use the interactive data).

[114] IBID

[115] Population Division of the Department of Economic and Social Affairs of the United Nations Secretariat, World Population Prospects: Esa.unorg 2017.

[116] Haiti by the numbers 2015: (https://haitipartners.org/haiti-statistics)

[117] COVID-19 is Spiking in Haiti. Can We Trust the Numbers? https:// www.newsweek.com/covid-19-spiking-haiti-can-we-trust-numbers-opinion-1601036

[118] Conspiracy Theories, Misinformation Abound as Haitians Brace for Coronavirus. https://www.voanews.com/science-health/coronavirus-outbreak/conspiracy-theories-misinformation-abound-haitians-brace.

[119] Haiti: Between denial and fears about COVID-19, health promotion on the front line. Retrieved from https://

www.reliefweb.int/report/haiti/haiti-between-denial-and-fears-about-covid-19-health-promotion-front-line.

[120] (2020). Dying to live: Haiti's COVID-19 paradox. Harvard International Review, https://hir.harvard.edu/haitis-covid-19-paradox/

[121] USVI COVID-19 Timeline, The Government of the United States Virgin Islands. Retrieved from https://www.vi.gov/usvi-covid-19-timeline/

[122] Haiti needs a strong COVID-19 response to maintain national stability | | UN News; retrieved from https://news.un.org/en.story/2020/06/1066752

[123] COVID-19 in Haiti - The Current Response and Challenges. Retrieved from https://cepr.net/covid-19-in-haiti-the-current-response-and-challenges

[124] As Haiti Braces for the COVID-19 Pandemic, Water, Sanitation, and Hygiene Are More Important Than Ever. Retrieved from https://www.worldbank.org/en/news/feature/2020/05/29/as-haiti-braces-for-the-covid-19-pandemic-water-sanitation-and-hygiene-are-more-important-than-ever

[125] Texas Lt. Governor: Old People Should Volunteer to Die to Save the Economy; Vanity Fair online; https://www.vanityfair.com/news/2020/03/dan-patrick-coronavirus-grandparents

[126] Swift, Jim; (2020). The "Let the Elderly Die' chorus; Retrieved from https://thebulwark.com/the-let-the-elderly-die-chorus/

[127] Italy's large elderly population bearing brunt of coronavirus. Retrieved from https://www.theguardian.com/world/2020/mar/03/italy-elderly-population-coronavirus-risk-covid-19

[128] Supporting older people during the COVID-19 pandemic is everyone's business: https://www.euro.who.int/en/health-topics/health-emergencies/coronavirus-covid-19/news/news/2020/4/supporting-older-people-during-the-covid-19-pandemic-is-everyones-business

[129] If You Are Immunocompromised, Protect Yourself From COVID 19:https://www.cdc.gov/coronavirus/2019-ncov/need-extra precautions/immunocompromised.html

[130] WHO Coronavirus Disease (COVID-19) Dashboard: https://covid19.who.int.

[131] Explained: These are the countries that have not imposed lockdowns. Retrieved from https://indianexpress.com/article/explained-the-countries-that-have-not-imposed-lockdowns-and-why-6389003

[132] Felter, C. & Bussemaker, N. (2020). Which countries are requiring face masks? Retrieved from https://www.cfr.org/in-brief/which-coountries-are-requiring-face3-masks

[133] Coronavirus 2019 disease (COVID-19): COVID-19 Myths and Misconceptions

[134] The U.S. Surgeon General is calling COVID-19 misinformation an 'urgent threat'.
Retrieved from https://www.npr.org/sections/health-shots/2021/07/15/1016013826/the-u-s-surgeon-general-is-calling-covid-19-misinformation-an-urgent-threat

[135] COVID-19 and Psychological denial (2020): https://www.cjshane.com/blog/the-world-covid-19-and-psychological-denial.TheAmerican Psychological Association

[136] Child Development: Ages and Stages https://www.choc.org/primary-care/ages-stages

[137] Denying the reality of the coronavirus has made it more dangerous for everyone. https://www.nbcnews.com/think/opinion/denying-reality-coronavirus-has-made-it-more-dangerous-everyone-ncna1175916

[138] Melinda gates: 'Every life has equal value.' Retrieved from https://www.thelily.com/melinda-gates-every-life-has-equal-value/

[139] Every Life Has Equal Value. Retrieved from https://www.sciencedirect.com/science/article/pii/S0092867413010775

[140] WHO Coronavirus Disease (COVID-19) Dashboard: https://covid19.who.int.

[141] Advice on the use of masks in COVID-19 https://www.who.int/emergencies/diseases/novel-coronavirus-2019/advice-for-public/when-and-how-to-use-masks

[142] Considerations for Wearing Cloth Face Coverings: https://www.cdc.gov/coronavirus/2019-ncov/prevent-getting-sick/cloth-face-cover-guidance.

[143] IBID

[144] Here is Why the CDC's New COVID-19 Guidelines Urge You to Wear a Mask: https://Heavy.com/news/2020/07/covid-19-masks-cdc.

[145] Considerations for Wearing Cloth Face Coverings:https://www.cdc.gov/coronavirus/2019-ncov/prevent-getting-sick/cloth-face-cover-guidance.html.

[146] Here is Why the CDC's New COVID-19 Guidelines Urge You to Wear a Mask: https://Heavy.com/news/2020/07/COVID-19-masks-cdc.

[147] (2020). As many as 130,000 lives could be saved in the next 3 months if everyone wore a mask. Retrieved from https://www.healthline.com/health-news/as-many-as-130000-lives-could-be-saved-the-next-3-months-if-everyone-wore-a-mask

[148] (2020). COVID-19 Cough Test – Without mask vs. with mask vs. with hand Retrieved from https://www.youtube.com/watch?v=b4ts7VflPno

[149} IBID

[150] (2020). Best masks to keep COVID-19 to yourself. Retrieved from https://www.youtube.com/watch?v=RkB0k81oNiI

[151] High speed camera captures how different types of face masks work: Face covering and mask to minimize droplet dispersion and aerosolization. Retrieved fromhttps://www.youtube.com/watch?v=DNeYfUTA11s

[152] (2020). Researchers test mask using coronavirus. Retrieved from https://www.youtube.com/watch?v=3GndKYJ4uBI

[153] (2021). Talking spreads COVID far more than coughing or sneezing, study concludes. Retrieved from https://www.studyfinds.org/talking-spreads-covid-more-than-coughing-sneezing

[154] (2020). Trump says masks area 'double-edged sword.' Goldman Sachs says they could help save the economy. Retrieved from https://www.cnn.com/2020/06/30/business/face-masks-economic-recovery-goldman-sachs/index.html

[155] WHO Coronavirus Disease (COVID-19) Dashboard https://covid19.who.int.

[156] Orbert, Jessica;(2021). Haiti still awaiting first COVID vaccines, as cases surge. Retrieved from https://haitiantimes.com/2021/07/06/haiti-still-awaiting-first-covid-vaccines-as-cases-surge/

[157] (2020, May). Why Africa struggles to test for COVID-19; Retrieved from https://www.economist.com/graphic-detail/2020/05/26/why-africa-struggles-to-test-for-covid-19

[158] Statistics re: numbers of tests performed to date (July2021) in the African Continent; Retrieved from https://africacdc.org/covid-19/

[159] Statistics re: numbers of tests performed to date (July 2021) in the USVI retrieved from https://covidusa.net/?state=Virgin+Islands

[160] (2021). Experts puzzeled by why Haiti has one of the lowest COVID-19 death rates in the world despite administering zero vaccine doses: We Don't Know. Retrieved from https://atlantablackstar.com/2021/05/11/experts-puzzled-by-why-haiti-has-one-of-the-lowest-covid-19-death-rates-in-the-world-despite-administering-zero-vaccine-doses-we-dont-know/

[161] (2020). Behind the COVID numbers in Haiti. Retrieved from https://nacla.org/news/2020/06/09/behind-covid-numbers-haiti

[162] (2020). African countries conduct over 8.3 mln COVID-19tests amid rapid infection rate: Africa CDC; retrieved from https://africa.cgtn.com/2020/07/29/african-countries-conduct-over-8-3-mln-covid-19-tests-amid-rapid-infection-rate-africa-cdc/

[163] Before Vaccines, Doctors 'Borrowed' Antibodies from Recovered Patients to Save Lives. https://www.history.com/news/blood-plasma-covid-19-measles-spanish-flu

[164] Potential Use of Convalescent Plasma During a Flu Pandemic. https//www.who.int/medicines/areas/quality_safety/regulation_legislation/icdra/5_USA_ConvalescentPlasmaDuringPandemic.pdf?ua=1

[165] Convalescent plasma therapy - a silver lining for COVID-19 management? Published online 2021 Apr 21. doi: 10.1016/j.htct.2021.03.004. https://www.ncbi.nlm.nih.gov/pmc/articles/PMC8059940/

[166] WHO lists two COVID-19 tests for emergency use: https://www.who.int/news-room/detail/07-04-2020-who-lists-two-covid-19-tests-for-emergency-use

[167] Antibodies protect against COVID-19 Reinfection; retrieved from https://newsinhealth.nih.gov/2021/04/antibodies-protect-against-covid-19-reinfection

[168] Good News: Mild COVID-19induces lasting antibody protection; retrieved from https://medicine.wustl.edu/news/good-news-mild-covid-19-induces-lasting-antibody-protection/

[169] SARS=CoV-2 Antibodies can protect from reinfection, NCI study suggests; retrieved from https://www.cancer.gov/news-events/cancer-currents-blog/2020/coronavirus-antibodies-protect-against-future-infection

[170] What you should know about antibody testing; retrieved from https://health.howstuffworks.com/human-body/systems/immune/antibody-testing.htm

[171] Antibody (Serology) testing for COVID-19: Information for patients and consumers; retrieved from https://www.fda.gov/medical-devices/coronavirus-covid-19-and-medical-devices/antibody-serology-testing-covid-

19-information-patients-and-consumers

[172] Not all coronavirus patients develop COVID -19 antibodies, study finds; retrieved from https://www.independent.co.uk/news/health/coronavirus-antibody-test-covid-19-a9567171.html

[173] An infodemic definition: https://www.Dictionary.com/e/pop-culture/infodemic

[174] UN tackles "infodemic" of misinformation and cybercrime in COVID-19 crisis; retrieved from https://www.un.org/en/un-coronavirus-communications-team/un-tackling-%E2%80%98infodemic%E2%80%99-misinformation-and-cybercrime-covid-19

[175] COVID-19: Social media users more likely to believe false information; retrieved from https://www.mcgill.ca/newsroom/channels/news/covid-19-social-media-users-more-likely-believe-false-information-323390

[176] Americans are super-spreaders of COVID-19 misinformation, retrieved from https://www.mcgill.ca/newsroom/channels/news/americans-are-super-spreaders-covid-19-misinformation-330229

[177] Busari S, Adebayo B. Nigeria records chloroquine poisoning after Trump endorses it for coronavirus treatment; retrieved from https://edition.cnn.com/2020/03/23/africa/chloroquine-trump-nigeria-intl/index.html

[178] Kasulis K. Patient 31 and South Korean's sudden spike in coronavirus cases. Alijazeera; 2020: https://www.aljazeera.com/news/2020/3/3/patient-31-and-south-koreas-sudden-spike-in-coronavirus-cases.

[179] Statt N. Major tech platforms say they are jointly combating fraud and misinformation 'about COVID-19. Verge;2020; retrieved from https://www.theverge.com/2020/3/16/21182726/coronavirus-covid-19-facebook-google-twitter-youtube-joint-efforts-misinformation-fraud

[180] Basch CH, Basch CE, Ruggles KV, Hammond R. Coverage of the Ebola Virus Disease Epidemic on YouTube. Disaster Med Public Health Prep. 2015 Oct;9(5):531-5. doi: 10.1017/dmp.2015.77. Epub 2015 Jun 19. PMID: 26088275.

[181] Shu K, Sliva A, Wang S, Tang J, Liu H. Fake news detection on social media: a data mining perspective,

2017; retrieved from https://arxiv.org/abs/1708.01967

[182] HK police arrest man "for spreading fake news" RTHK News; 2020: https://news.rthk.hk/rthk/en/component/k2.

[183] Lagosians complain of hunger only days into coronavirus lockdown, retrieved from https://www.pulse.ng/news/local/coronavirus-lagosians-complain-of-hunger-only-days-into-lockdown/15sw6tj

[184] Uganda's urban poor fear dying of hunger during COVID-19; retrieved from https://allianceforscience.cornell.edu/blog/2020/04/ugandas-urban-poor-fear-dying-of-hunger-during-covid-19-lockdown/

[185] COVID pushes millions more children deeper into poverty, new study finds, retrieved from https://news.un.org/en/story/2020/09/1072602

[186] The devastating consequences of coronavirus lockdowns in poor countries, retrieved from https://www.vox.com/future-perfect/2020/4/18/21212688/coronavirus-lockdowns-developing-world

[187] As hunger rises, Philippine authorities take aim at

farmers and rural activists; retrieved from https://www.thenewhumanitarian.org/news/2021/4/20/food-hunger-and-covid-19-in-the-philippines

[188] Pandemic policies in poor places; retrieved from https://www.cgdev.org/publication/pandemic-policies-poor-places

[189] Hunger stalks India's poor in COVID-19 pandemic double blow; retrieved from https://www.channelnewsasia.com/news/asia/india-covid-19-pandemic-hunger-poverty-economic-crisis-14914348

[190] Cambodians complain of lockdown hunger as outbreak takes toll on poor; retrieved from https://www.reuters.com/world/asia-pacific/cambodians-complain-lockdown-hunger-outbreak-takes-toll-poor-2021-04-30/

[191] Employment in Africa: Think agriculture: https://www.ilo.org/global/about-the-ilo/newsroom/news/WCMS_203469/langen/index.htm

[192] Across Africa, a reliance on the informal sector threatens effective coronavirus lockdowns; retrieved from https://qz.com/africa/1831785/coronavirus-citizens-

in-africas-informal-economy-try-to-survive.

[193] Five facts about the informal economy in Africa; retrieved from https://www.ilo.org/africa/whats-new/WCMS_377286/lang--en/index.html.

[194] Haiti's informal economy complicates efforts to fight pandemic; retrieved from https://www.americamagazine.org/politics-society/2020/03/26/haitis-informal-economy-complicates-efforts-fight-pandemic

[195] Dying to Live: Haiti's COVID-19 paradox; retrieved from https://hir.harvard.edu/haitis-covid-19-paradox/

[196] Haiti population clash with police for hunger; retrieved from https://www.bing.com/videos/search/Haiti+population+hunger+clas+with+police+fbeor+hunger.

[197] Protest in Haiti Over Hunger and Repressive Rule; retrieved from https://stephenlendman.org/2019/02/protests-in-haiti-over-hunger-and-repressive-rule/.

[198] The Politics of Crackdowns on Africa's Informal

Vendors: https://www.ingentaconnect.com/content/cuny/cp/2019/

[199] Policy Responses To COVID-19: https://www.imf.org/en/Topics/imf-and-covid19/Policy-Responses-to-COVID-19.

[200] Coronavirus: Nigeria seeks a $7bn loan from international lenders: https://www.theafricareport.com/25762/coronavirus-nigeria-seeks-6-9bn-loan-from-international-lenders

[201] Africa in the news: New-Africa strategy, impacts of the oil price crash, and spread of coronavirus. Retrieved from https://www.brookings.edu/blog/africa-in-focus/2020/03/14/africa-in-the-news-new-eu-africa-strategy-impacts-of-the-oil-price-crash-and-spread-of-coronavirus.

[202] Bold steps to pump coronavirus rescue funds down the last mile: https://www.ft.com/content/5a1a1e9c-6f4d-11ea-89df-41bea055720b.

[203] Amstrong, D. & Griffin, R. (2020). COVID-19 shaping up to be battle for years even with Vaccine. Retrieved from https://www.bloomberg.com/news/

articles/2020-08-13/get-used-to-living-with-covid-19-for-a-long-time-experts-say

[204] Pratt, Elizabeth, (2020). COVID-19 could become a seasonal illness: What we'll need to do. Retrieved from https://www.healthline.com/health-news/covid19-could-become-seasonal-just-like-the-flu

[205] Freedman, A. & Samenow, J. (2020). Coronavirus may have a seasonal cycle, but that doesn't mean it will go away this summer, experts warn. Retrieved from https://www.washingtonpost.com/weather/2020/03/11/coronavirus-may-have-seasonal-cycle-that-doesnt-mean-it-will-go-away-this-summer-experts-warn/

[206] Jeffrey Shaman, Edward Goldstein, Marc Lipsitch, Absolute Humidity and Pandemic Versus Epidemic Influenza, American Journal of Epidemiology, Volume 173, Issue 2, 15 January 2011, Pages 127–135, https://doi.org/10.1093/aje/kwq347 Retrieved from https://academic.oup.com/aje/article/173/2/127/99316

[207] Freedman, A. & Samenow, J. (2020). Coronavirus may have a seasonal cycle, but that doesn't mean it will go away this summer, experts warn. Retrieved from https://www.washingtonpost.com/weather/2020/03/11/

coronavirus-may-have-seasonal-cycle-that-doesnt-mean-it-will-go-away-this-summer-experts-warn/

[208] Jeffrey Shaman, Edward Goldstein, Marc Lipsitch, Absolute Humidity and Pandemic Versus Epidemic Influenza, American Journal of Epidemiology, Volume 173, Issue 2, 15 January 2011, Pages 127–135, https://doi.org/10.1093/aje/kwq347
Retrieved from https://academic.oup.com/aje/article/173/2/127/99316

[209] IBID

[210] McKim, Claire, (2020). Edinburgh University professor Devi Sridhar: Inevitable now that England will see a rise in cases. Retrieved from https:// www.edinburghlive.co.uk/news/edinburgh-news/edinburgh-university-professor-devi-sridhar-18337838

[211] Experts predict what life will be like after a COVID-19 vaccine arrives. Retrieved from https://www.huffpost.com/entry/life-after-covid-19-vaccine_l_5f2ad9c6c5b64d7a55ed7b2c

[212] Morbidity and Mortality Weekly Report (MMWR): https://www.cdc.gov/mmwr/volumes/69/wr/mm6912e2.htm

[213] Whitehouse, David (2020). Africa needs more health data to improve response to health crises; (2020). Retrieved from https://www.theafricareport.com/25951/lack-of-statistical-capacity-means-africa-risks-shooting-in-the-dark-on-coronavirus/

[214] Morbidity and Mortality Weekly Report (MMWR): https://www.cdc.gov/mmwr/volumes/69/wr/mm6912e2.htm.

[215] WHO: access to HIV medicines severely impacted by COVID-19 as AIDS response stalls: https://www.who.int/news-room/detail/06-07-2020-who-access-to-hiv-medicines-severely-impacted-by-COVID-19-as-aids-response-stalls

[216] Cancer Screening During the COVID-19 Pandemic. Retrieved from https://www.cancer.org/healthy/find-cancer-early/cancer-screening-guidelines/cancer-screening-during-covid-19-pandemic.html

[217] NAFDAC confirms the use of chloroquine for COVID-19 treatment. Retrieved from https://www.ripplesnigeria.com/nafdac-confirms-use-of-chloroquine-for-covid-19-treatment

[218] WHO pauses the study of hydroxychloroquine in the global trial. Retrieved from https://www.politico.eu/article/who-pauses-study-of-hydroxychloroquine-in-global-trial.

[219] The FDA warns against the widespread use of hydroxychloroquine. Retrieved from https://www.statnews.com/2020/04/24/fda-warns-against-widespread-use-of-hydroxychloroquine-drug-touted-by-trump

[220] France bans the use of hydroxychloroquine as coronavirus treatment. Retrieved from https://www.politico.com/news/2020/05/27/france-bans-use-of-hydroxychloroquine-to-cure-coronavirus.

[221] COVID in Africa; retrieved from https://news.sky.com/story/covid-19-in-africa-why-is-the-death-rate-so-low-12236347

[222] IBID

[223] https://www.worldometers.info/coronavirus/country/haiti/

[224] https://covidusa.net/?autorefresh=1&state=Virgin+Islands

[225] https://allafrica.com/view/group/main/main/id/00072212.html

[226] (2021). COVID-19 kills over 156,000 in Africa as cases surge to 6 M. Retrieved from https://healthwise.punchng.com/covid-19-kills-over-156000-in-africa-as-cases-surge-to-6m/

[227] COVID-19: New variants in Africa spark concern; retrieved from https://www.msn.com/en-xl/africa/other/covid-19-new-variants-in-africa-spark-concern/ar-AAKfLCd

[228] IBID

[229] IBID

[230] CDC: About 5,800 fully vaccinated people have tested positive for COVID-19; retrieved from https://www.msn.com/en-us/health/medical/cdc-about-5800-fully-vaccinated-people-have-tested-positive-for-covid-19/ar-BB1fHfC1

[231] So far, 5,800 fully vaccinated people have caught COVID anyway in US, CDC says; retrieved from https://www.cnn.com/2021/04/14/health/breakthrough-

infections-covid-vaccines-cdc/index.html

[232] Learning from the. Best: Evaluating Africa's COVID-19 responses; retrieved from https://www.brookings.edu/blog/africa-in-focus/2020/07/08/learning-from-the-best-evaluating-africas-covid-19-responses/

[233] IBID

[234] Roll out of rapid testing could be a 'game changer' for Africa; retrieved from https://www.devex.com/news/roll-out-of-rapid-testing-could-be-a-game-changer-for-africa-98386

[235] IBID

[236] IBID

[237] IBID

[238] City Reaches Milestone of Testing 20,000 New Yorkers Per Day and Triples Number of Available Testing Sites with City MD; retrieved from https://www1.nyc.gov/office-of-the-mayor/news/351-20/city-reaches-milestone-testing-20-000-new-yorkers-day-triples-number-available

[239] Lack of Covid-19 testing undermines Africa's success; retrieved from https://www.bbc.com/news/world-africa.

[240] Testing Kits in Africa Deemed Faulty After COVID-19 Confirmed in Goat, Quail, Pawpaw; retrieved from https://www.cnsnews.com/article/international/patrick-goodenough/testing-kits-africa-deemed-faulty-after-covid-19-confirmed.

[241] IBID

[242] WHO ramps up COVID-19 support to hotspot countries in Africa; retrieved from https://www.afro.who.int/news/who-ramps-COVID-19-support-hotspot-countries-africa.

[243] Movie theaters may pose less COVID-19 risk than we think, says UC Davis Health Expert. Retrieved from https:// health.ucdavis.edu/health-news/newsroom/movie-theaters-may-pose-less-covid19-risk-than-we-think-says-uc-davis-health-expert/2020/06.

[244] Requirement for face masks on public transportation conveyances and transportation hubs. Retrieved from https: www.cdc.gov/coronavirus/2019-ncov/travelers/face-masks-public-transportation.html

[245] (2021). Fact checks: How safe is flying during the COVID pandemic? Retrieved from https://www.dw.com/en/how-safe-is-flying-during-the-covid-pandemic/a-57284835

[246] Bushwick, S.; Lewis, L.; Montanex, A. (2020). Evaluating COVID risk on planes, trains, and automobiles. https://www.scientificamerican.com/article/evaluating-covid-risk-on-planes-trains-and-automobiles2/

[247] Why are places of worship so susceptible to COVID-19 outbreaks? Retrieved from https://www.today.com/health/why-are-places-worship-so-susceptible-covid-19-outbreaks-t188095

[248] Bierer, B. E., White, S. A., Barnes, J. M., & Gelinas, L. (2020). Ethical Challenges in Clinical Research During the COVID-19 Pandemic. Journal of bioethical inquiry, 17(4), 717–722. https://doi.org/10.1007/s11673-020-10045-4
Retrieved from https://www.ncbi.nlm.nih.gov/pmc/articles/PMC7651825/

[249] Lai CC, Shih TP, Ko WC, et al. Severe acute respiratory syndrome coronavirus 2 (SARS-CoV-2) and coronavirus disease-2019 (COVID-19): the epidemic and challenges.

https://www.cmaj.ca/content/192/15/E405

[250] Matthew P. Cheng, Todd C. Lee, Darrell H.S. Tan and Srinivas Murthy (2020). Generating randomized trial evidence to optimize treatment in the COVID-19 pandemic.
CMAJ April 14, 2020, 192 (15) E405-E407; DOI: https://doi.org/10.1503/cmaj.200438. Retrieved from https://www.cmaj.ca/content/192/15/E405

[251] IBID

[252] COVID-19: The CIDRAP Viewpoint; retrieved from https://www.cidrap.umn.edu/sites/default/files/public/downloads/cidrap-covid19-viewpoint-part1_0.pdf.

[253] The expert report predicts up to two more years of pandemic misery; retrieved from https://www.cnn.com/2020/04/30/health/report-covid-two-more-years/index.html

[254] CDC: Asymptomatic carriers make up 40% of people infected with coronavirus. Retrieved from https://www.kron4.com/health/coronavirus/cdc-asymptomatic-carriers-make-up-40-of-people-infected-with-coronavirus/.

[255] The expert report predicts up to two more years of pandemic misery. Retrieved from https://www.cnn.com/2020/04/30/health/report-covid-two-more-years/index.html.

[256] Jonathan Smith, Epidemiology of Microbial Diseases and Global Health at Yale
University School of Public Health (2020). 'I Promise. I Promise.' You Can't Cheat A
Pandemic; retrieved from https://www.wbur.org/cognoscenti/2020/04/03/hold-the-line-
coronavirus-Jonathan-smith

[257] Trace Together app becomes primary tracking tool and compulsory in many
settings. retrieved from
https://www.theregister.com/2021/05/17/singapore_changes_covid_tracking_tech/

[258] Tracing surveillance and auto-regulation in Singapore: 'smart' responses to COVID-
19 retrieved from https://journals.sagepub.com/doi/full/10.1177/1329878X20949545/
https://doi.org/10.1177/1329878X20949545

[259] (2020). Over 70 million people expected to fall into

extreme poverty due to COVID-19. Retrieved from https://africa.cgtn.com/2020/07/08/over-70-million-people-expected-to-fall-into-extreme-poverty-due-to-COVID-19.

[260] (2020). UNECA projects COVID-19 could push 29 million Africans into extreme poverty. Retrieved from https://africa.cgtn.com/2020/06/04/uneca-projects-COVID-19-could-push-29-million-africans-into-extreme-poverty.

[261] Eames, Fine, and Heymann, "Herd immunity': A rough guide," pp. 911–6; retrieved from https://www.mckinsey.com/industries/healthcare-systems-and-services/our-insights/when-will-the-covid-19-pandemic-end.

[262] COVID-19 Delta variant to dominate other strains within months; retrieved from https://www.livemint.com/news/world/covid19-delta-variant-to-dominate-other-strains-within-months-says-who-11626871682857.html

[263] Miriam Berger, "U.K. variant continues to spread around the world as coronavirus pandemic enters 2021," Washington Post, Jan 2, 2021, washingtonpost.com.

[264] Carl Zimmer, "U.S. is blind to contagious new virus variant, scientists warn," *New York* Times, January 6, 2021, nytimes.com.

[265] Eric Volz et al., Transmission of SARS-CoV-2 Lineage B.1.1.7 in England: Insights from linking epidemiological and genetic data, Imperial College London, December 2020, imperial. ac. the UK.

[266] Nicholas Davies et al., Estimated transmissibility, and severity of novel SARS-CoV-2 Variant of Concern 202012/01 in England, Center for Mathematical Modeling of Infectious Diseases, December 2020, cmmid.github.io.

[267] COVID-19 Delta variant to dominate other strains within months; retrieved from https:// www.livemint.com/news/world/covid19-delta-variant-to-dominate-other-strains-within-months-says-who-11626871682857.html

[268] COVID-19 Delta variant to dominate other strains within Months; retrieved from https:// www.livemint.com/ news/world/covid19-delta-variant-to-dominate-other-strains-within-months-says-who-11626871682857.html

[269] IBID

[270] The effects of virus variants on COVID-19 vaccines; retrieved from https://www.who.int/news- room/feature-stories/detail/the-effects-of-virus-variants-on-covid-19-vaccines

[271] Haiti - COVID-19: Haiti is still not ready to receive vaccines, June 2021; retrieved from https://www.haitilibre.com/en/news-33656-haiti-covid-19-haiti-is-still-not-ready-to-receive-vaccines.html

[272] Haiti is the only country in the western hemisphere without vaccines. June 8, 2021. retrieved from https://www.bloomberg.com/news/articles/2021-06-08/haiti-is-the-only-country-in-western-hemisphere-without-vaccines

[273] Haiti receives 500,000 vaccines donated by the United States through COVAX; JULY 14,2021; retrieved from https://www.paho.org/en/news/14-7-2021-haiti-receives-500000-vaccines-donated-united-states-through-covax

[274] The effects of virus variants on COVID-19 vaccines.

Vaccines Explained series;
retrieved from https://www.who.int/news-room/feature-stories/detail/the-effects-of- virus-variants-on-covid-19-vacc

[275] Another study finds cross-reactivity T cell responses against SARS-CoV-2; retrieved
from https://www.news-medical.net/news/20201005/Another-study-finds-cross-reactivity-T-cell-responses-against-SARS-CoV-2.aspx

[276] SARS-CoV-2 immunity: review and applications to phase 3 vaccine candidates Published
online 2020 Oct 13. doi: 10.1016/S0140-6736(20)32137-1; retrieved from https://www.ncbi.nlm.nih.gov/pmc/articles/PMC7553736/

[277] WHO Key criteria for the ethical acceptability of COVID-19 human challenge studies. May 6, 2020. Retrieved from https://apps.who.int/iris/bitstream/handle/10665/331976/WHO-2019-nCoV-Ethics_criteria-2020.1-eng.pdf?ua=1 [Ref list]

APPENDIX A

Also, by Dr. Hugues F. Batsielilit, Ph.D.

False-Positive HIV Test Results: The Silent Issue in African Countries

This first book was prompted by the disregard for the increasing impact false-positive results have on individuals and communities resulting in an overall failure in the confidence Africans have for battling the soaring negative impacts of HIV. It can be purchased by visiting the link provided below:

https://books2read.com/u/47OwdN

Telemedicine Services: An Argument for Use in Africa, Haiti, and the U.S. Virgin Islands Healthcare Systems

This second book examines the benefits of Telemedicine against the backdrop of the reality that existing systems are deficient, not prioritized by the governments, and people - especially those residing in rural areas - are suffering, even dying. Telemedicine technology can help repair and expand these broken health systems and bring critical health services to those most in need. It can be purchased by visiting the link provided below:

https://books2read.com/u/bOJweA

APPENDIX B

Don't Miss Out!

Dr. Hugues F Batsielilit, Ph.D. is an avid writer and researcher. You do not want to miss out on any his new material so please go to the link provided below to sign up for notifications whenever he publishes a new book. There is no charge or obligation for doing so.

https://books2read.com/r/B-A-FYGP-SSRSB

Made in the USA
Monee, IL
05 November 2026

67845292R00138